Pharynx - The Incredible Rendezvous Sites of Gas, Liquid and Solid

Edited by Tang-Chuan Wang

Published in London, United Kingdom

Pharynx - The Incredible Rendezvous Sites of Gas, Liquid and Solid
http://dx.doi.org/10.5772/intechopen.98063
Edited by Tang-Chuan Wang

Contributors
Subramaniam Vinayak, Mohak Kumar, Oancea Alina Lavinia Antoaneta, Berteşteanu Şerban Vifor Gabriel, Grigore Raluca, Popescu Bogdan, Suhaib A.H AL-Taai, Michael Stevens, Paula Luiza Bejenaru, Raluca Grigore, Alexandru Nicolaescu, Mihnea Cojocarita-Condeescu, Catrinel Simion-Antonie, Gloria Munteanu, Anca Cirstea, Teodora Diaconu, Bianca Taher, Simona Rujan, Dan Popescu, Tang-Chuan Wang

First published in London, United Kingdom, 2022 by IntechOpen
IntechOpen is the global imprint of INTECHOPEN LIMITED, registered in England and Wales, registration number: 11086078, 5 Princes Gate Court, London, SW7 2QJ, United Kingdom

British Library Cataloguing-in-Publication Data
A catalogue record for this book is available from the British Library

Additional hard and PDF copies can be obtained from orders@intechopen.com

Pharynx - The Incredible Rendezvous Sites of Gas, Liquid and Solid
Edited by Tang-Chuan Wang
p. cm.
Print ISBN 978-1-80355-195-1
Online ISBN 978-1-80355-196-8
eBook (PDF) ISBN 978-1-80355-197-5

Meet the editor

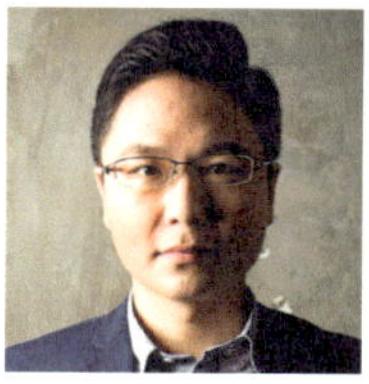

Dr. Tang-Chuan Wang is an otolaryngologist and head and neck surgeon in Taiwan. He is also a research scholar at Harvard Medical School and the University of Iowa hospital. He has extensive work experience in the United States, including at Stanford University, the University of Pennsylvania, Boston Children's Hospital, and Massachusetts Eye and Ear. In addition to clinical and basic medicine, Dr. Wang is interested in public health. In recent years, he has devoted his time to innovation and telemedicine. Due to his contribution to biodesign, he was invited to join the executive committee of the Metal Industries R & D Center, Taiwan.

Contents

Preface

The pharynx is an incredible structure in the human body. The pharynx is a conical passage connecting the oral cavity and nasal cavity to the junction of the esophagus and trachea. There is also another passage called the eustachian or pharyngotympanic tube, which links the nasopharynx to the middle ear.

The pharynx moves food or water from the mouth to the esophagus and moves air from the nasal and oral cavities to the larynx. The larynx, the nearby structure, is a triangle-shaped box that consists largely of cartilages with surrounding structures, including muscles, fibers, and elastic tissue components. They play important roles in swallowing, breathing, producing sound, and protecting the trachea against food aspiration. During the normal speech, air comes from the lungs and sound comes from the vocal cords and then travels upward in the pharynx. In other words, the pharynx is a dynamic rendezvous site of gases (air), liquids (water), and solids (food).

Although the pharynx is relatively small compared to other organ systems, it is just as vital. For example, obstructive sleep apnea, the most common sleep-related breathing disorder, is characterized by repetitive collapse and closing of the pharynx during sleep. The most common cause of sleep apnea in children is enlarged tonsils and adenoids that block the airway and obstruct breathing during sleep. In addition, there are some conditions that can cause the pharynx to not function properly, affecting digestion, respiration, phonation, or sleep.

The pharynx is a crossroad in the upper part of the digestive and respiratory pathways and malignancy at this level leads to the impairment of vital functions, such as breathing, feeding, and speech. Pharyngeal cancer is one of the most challenging cancers in terms of location, evolution, prognosis, and functional implications. With advances in treatment, surgery and reconstruction techniques can deliver an adequate quality of life for patients. Pharyngeal reconstruction is a complex and difficult process that should involve a combined evaluation of the size and location of the defect, the patient's age and comorbid status, and the simplest reconstruction with the greatest level of function.

Based on these concepts, the book highlights developments as well as future perspectives in the ever-expanding field of pharynx health. It is a great reference for otolaryngologists, pulmonologists, gastroenterologists, pediatricians, neurologists, and other medical professionals.

I am grateful to everyone who has contributed to the editorial process of this book, including the wonderful staff at IntechOpen. This book would not be possible without their help and support. I would also like to express my gratitude to my family, teachers, and colleagues.

Tang-Chuan Wang
Chairman of Otolaryngology-Head and Neck Surgery,
China Medical University Hsinchu Hospital,
Taiwan

School of Medicine,
College of Medicine,
China Medical University,
Taiwan

Department of Biomedical Engineering,
College of Biomedical Engineering,
China Medical University,
Taiwan

Research Scholar of Harvard Medical School,
MA, USA

Research Scholar of University of Iowa Hospitals and Clinics,
IA, USA

Member of American Academy of Otolaryngology-Head and Neck Surgery

Fellow of the American College of Surgeons

Section 1

Introduction - The Incredible Pharynx Affecting Human Life

Chapter 1

Introductory Chapter: Pharynx - The Important Role Involved in Both Respiratory and Digestive Systems

Tang-Chuan Wang

1. Introduction

The pharynx is a special structure in the human body. Pharynx is a conical passage connecting the oral cavity and nasal cavity to the junction of the esophagus and trachea. Besides, there is another passage, called Eustachian tube or pharyngotympanic tube, which links the nasopharynx to the middle ear and it allows air pressure in the middle ear cavity to be equalized. The pharynx moves food or water from the mouth to the esophagus and also moves air from the nasal and oral cavities to the larynx. Therefore, the pharynx plays an important role involved in both the respiratory and digestive systems. In other words, the pharynx is an incredibly dynamic rendezvous site of gas(air), liquid(water), and solid(food).

2. Functional pharynx affects human basic life

Although the pharynx is relatively small compared to other organ systems, a person's basic life will be affected greatly without well functional pharynx. For example, obstructive sleep apnea syndrome, the most common sleep-related breathing disorder, is characterized by repetitive collapse and closing of the pharynx during sleep. The most common cause of sleep apnea in children is enlarged tonsils and adenoids that block the airway and interrupt breathing during sleep. The recurrent episodes of apneas or hypopneas during sleep may interfere with restorative sleep in combination with disturbances in blood oxygenation. And these are possible negative consequences to health and quality of life. Upper airway image analysis may be helpful for these patients. Neck CT with computational fluid dynamics study is good for evaluating airway pressure and airflow velocity, especially on obstructive sleep apnea syndrome. Besides, there are some disorders that can cause pharynx and larynx to not function properly, such as digestion, respiration, or phonation.

3. Pharyngeal cancer: one of the most challenging cancers

Cancer is undoubtedly an important issue of modern medicine. Cancer is a disease in which some of the body's cells grow uncontrollably and spread to other parts of the body. Cancer can start almost anywhere in the human body, which is made up of trillions of cells. Pharyngeal cancer includes cancer of the nasopharynx, the oropharynx, and the hypopharynx. The pharynx is a crossroad in the upper part of digestive and respiratory pathways and malignant appearance at this level leads to the impairment of vital functions, such as breathing, feeding, and speech. Therefore, we can advocate that pharyngeal cancer is one of the most challenging cancers regarding location, evolution, prognosis, and functional implications. Even if pharyngeal malignancies usually present high rate of mortality, the standard treatments for pharyngeal cancer include one or a combination of surgery, radiation, and chemotherapy with various results depending on the cancer stage.

4. Pharyngeal reconstruction: to restore a better life

The standard treatments for pharyngeal cancer include one or a combination of surgery, radiation, and chemotherapy with various results depending on the stage. The anatomic structure of the treated site is usually altered due to the treatment. The alteration causes adverse effects depending on the location of the primary tumor. With treatment development, a variety of surgical skills and reconstruction techniques can deliver an adequate quality of life for the patients. Pharyngeal reconstruction is a complex and difficult process that should perform a combined evaluation of the size, location of the defect, patient's age and comorbid status, and the use of the simplest reconstruction with the highest level of function. Some authors of this book elaborated an algorithm with treatment choices for defects of the laryngopharynx, hypopharynx, and cervical esophagus. Anyway, it is important to restore a better life for patients.

5. Future perspectives in the field of pharynx

Based on these above concepts, the book incorporates updated developments as well as future perspectives in the ever-expanding field of pharynx. Besides, this book is also a great reference for otolaryngologists, pulmonologists, gastroenterologists, pediatricians, neurologists, rehabilitation physicians, speech-language pathologists, audiologists, specialists in sleep medicine, researchers in clinical and basic medicine, and experts in science and technology.

Conflict of interest

The author declare no conflict of interest.

Author details

Tang-Chuan Wang[1,2,3]

1 Department of Otolaryngology-Head and Neck Surgery, China Medical University Hsinchu Hospital, Taiwan

2 School of Medicine, College of Medicine, China Medical University, Taiwan

3 Department of Biomedical Engineering, College of Biomedical Engineering, China Medical University, Taiwan

*Address all correspondence to: tangchuan1020@gmail.com

Chapter 2

New Insights into Beethoven's Deafness

Michael Stevens

Abstract

There have been many theories proposed to explain the deafness of Ludwig van Beethoven, because his history is complex. Evidence of otosclerosis is lacking, because close gross examination of Beethoven's middle ear at autopsy did not find any otosclerotic foci. His slowly progressive hearing loss over a period of years differs from the reported cases of autoimmune hearing loss, which is rapidly progressive over a period of months. The absence of mercury in Beethoven's hair and bone samples leads us to conclude that his deafness was not due to syphilis, because in that era, syphilis was treated with mercury. Microscopic examination of bone samples and examination of the middle ear have found no evidence of Paget's Disease. High levels of lead found deep in the bone suggest repeated exposure over a long period of time. The finding of shrunken cochlear nerves at his autopsy is consistent with axonal degeneration due to heavy metals such as lead. Chronic low-level exposure, like Beethoven's, causes sensory and autonomic findings rather than the classic wrist drop due to motor neuropathy. Beethoven's physicians thought that he had alcohol dependence. He particularly liked wine to which lead had been added to improve the flavor. A live patient reported in 2021 from Italy with a slowly progressive hearing loss and other symptoms like Beethoven had, was found to have lead poisoning. Therefore, the most likely cause of Beethoven's deafness was his consumption of wine tainted with lead.

Keywords: lead, alcohol, otosclerosis autoimmune, syphilis, Paget's disease

1. Introduction

The reader may wonder why this chapter is part of a book about the pharynx. Although Beethoven had no problem with his pharynx, he did have problems with his ears and his gastrointestinal tract at both ends of the pharynx. The reason this is relevant is that new insights have come to light from information not available prior to this century. This has allowed a better picture of a problem that has been poorly understood for many years.

2. The eustachian tube

The pharynx, the incredible rendezvous site of gas, liquid, and solids, is connected in its superior aspect, or nasopharynx, to the ear *via* the eustachian tube. In its lower extension, it connects to the gastrointestinal tract posteriorly *via* the esophagus and anteriorly to the lungs *via* the larynx. The eustachian tube is a very interesting structure that is about 36 millimeters long. It is divided into two segments. The bony, nearest to the ear, comprises ⅓, and the cartilaginous, nearest to the nasopharynx, the other ⅔ of its length. The cartilaginous portion is part of the pharynx [1]. A popular misunderstanding is that the eustachian tube drains fluid from the ear, because it projects downward from the ear to the nasopharynx. However, its function is to ventilate the ear. The eustachian tube is normally closed. It opens with swallowing in response to the pull of the tensor and elevator veli palatini muscles. They are innervated by the pharyngeal plexus of the vagus nerve. When swallowing occurs, air from the nasopharynx goes up into the ear to maintain a balance of pressure between the closed cavity of the ear and the outside air. If the eustachian tube does not open, a negative pressure develops in the middle ear cavity that draws fluid from the mucus membrane into the middle ear cavity, resulting in a hearing loss.

Many things can impede the eustachian tube from opening. These include viral upper respiratory infections, such as the common cld, nasal allergies, and sinus infections. These cause swelling of the eustachian tube opening, preventing it from opening properly. These can be treated by decongestants, antihistamines, nasal steroids, and antibiotics. Adenoid hypertrophy or enlargement can block air getting into the ear and can be treated by surgery or adenoidectomy. Tumors, such as nasopharyngeal carcinoma that is common in people of oriental origin, can be treated by surgery, radiation, and chemotherapy.

In cases of chronic eustachian tube dysfunction that has not responded to conservative measures, fluid can be drained from the middle ear by means of a hole or myringotomy made in the tympanic membrane or ear drum. If the eustachian tube remains occluded, however, fluid will re-accumulate, because the tympanic membrane will heal in a few days. This will necessitate placement of a small tube through the tympanic membrane or tympanostomy, to allow air to enter the middle ear space so the fluid can reabsorb. In recent years, a new technique called eustachian tube dilation has been performed from either the middle ear [2] or the nasopharynx [3], to restore normal eustachian tube function.

3. A diagnostic dilemma

Beethoven had no problem with his eustachian tube, but he did have hearing loss, chronic gastrointestinal problems, intermittent pain in his extremities, depression, and alcohol dependence. There are many opinions regarding the etiology of Ludvig van Beethoven's hearing loss. This is due to lack of confirmatory evidence by present techniques such as hearing tests, radiological and blood studies. His overall medical history was also complex with many symptoms that lead to conflicting diagnosis. Two papers demonstrate this sharp difference of opinion that can be formed even about the same diagnosis.

One paper examined three fragments of what was felt to be "nearly with certainly" Beethoven's skull bone that did not show signs of Paget's disease and emphasized that "it must therefore be concluded that Beethoven's deafness was not caused by Paget's Osteitis Deformans" [4]. The other paper stated, thus Paget's disease, complicated by hyperparathyroidism, gout, and attempts to find relief of symptoms through the use of alcohol, quinine, and possibly salicylates, can explain virtually all of Beethoven's medical problems [5]. The title of the latter included: "A Pathologist Sounds a final Note."

Obviously, there is no final note sounded, given the opposite opinions formed by these authors. A major problem is the approach that physicians have used. In their search for a diagnosis, they try to fit Beethoven's multiple symptoms with a cause of hearing loss that they know little about and do not have personal experience with. This contrasts with the approach of someone familiar with causes of hearing loss making a diagnosis and then seeing if Beethoven's other problems can be explained by this diagnosis. Relevant literature regarding his hearing loss was critically examined and felt not to explain his loss. It was then discovered that by reexamining a previously considered diagnosis with current information, a diagnosis could be made that explained not only his hearing loss, but his other symptoms as well. This satisfied Ockham's razor, which is a principle of parsimony that postulates that among competing theories, the hypothesis with the fewest assumptions is the one best selected [6]. Although this principal does not apply in all cases where there are multiple symptoms, it does work here.

3.1 Approach to the dilemma

An extensive review of the musical and medical history of Beethoven's life was done as part of a master's degree in music history and literature at the University of Utah School of Music and is published in The Laryngoscope [7]. Literature subsequent to the publishing of that paper has also been critically examined to complete this chapter. All diagnoses of Beethoven's deafness previously considered are not reviewed in this chapter due to length constraints, but attention is given to those most compelling.

3.2 Important historical evidences

Although confirmatory evidence is not available, the history of his hearing loss is, available and reveals much regarding it. At 27 years of age, Beethoven first noticed a hearing problem with ringing in his ear and became aware that he missed words and phrases. He confessed this to a childhood friend and physician in a letter. He said, "for the last several years my hearing has grown weaker and weaker-I cannot hear the high notes of instruments or voices-I can hear sounds, but I cannot make out the words" [8]. His loss slowly and progressively got worse so that he stopped playing the piano in 1815. In 1822, he had to stop conducting. What does the history of his hearing loss tell us? First, it was slowly progressive over a period of years. Second, it involved the high frequencies, at least initially, and third, he had reduced discrimination. Reduced discrimination is often seen in individuals that have hearing loss in the high frequencies. This causes them to miss the consonant sounds of words, because consonant sounds involve high frequencies. They hear words, but do not understand them, because they hear the vowels that are largely composed of lower tones, but not the high-tone consonants that separate the vowels.

3.3 Otosclerosis

One of the popular theories regarding Beethoven's deafness is that of otosclerosis [9]. This is a disease that causes a slowly progressive loss and often begins in the teens or twenties like that experienced by Beethoven. However, people with otosclerosis usually do not have difficulty understanding words when the sounds are sufficiently loud. In other words, otosclerosis is usually associated with good discrimination. It is also inherited, and although it can skip several generations, it is striking that there is no history of hearing loss in Beethoven's musical family. The most significant feature against otosclerosis is that a close examination of his temporal bone, including the middle ear, at the time of his death, found no evidence of otosclerotic foci. These are white plaques that would have been easily seen by the naked eye. These would certainly have been present given the many years of his loss before death.

3.4 Autoimmune hearing loss

Autoimmune hearing loss has been described in association with autoimmune bowel disease, and since Beethoven had gastrointestinal problems, his hearing loss might be autoimmune [10, 11]. However, autoimmune hearing loss usually progresses rapidly over weeks or months often with accompanying episodes of vertigo. A review of the literature did not find any cases of autoimmune loss with such a slow progression like Beethoven's. In addition, autoimmune bowel disease is invariably accompanied by bloody diarrhea. Beethoven's loss was slowly progressive and lacked vertigo, and no bloody diarrhea was ever mentioned. At his autopsy, there were no adhesions, strictures, or perforations in the bowel that are seen with autoimmune bowel disease. This diagnosis therefore does not fit.

3.5 Syphilis

Another diagnosis suggested by a prominent otologist is acquired syphilis, because of the shrunken cochlear nerves found at autopsy [12]. However, none of Beethoven's 17 physicians considered the diagnosis of syphilis, and evaluation of Beethoven's hair and bone samples in 2000 and 2005 showed no evidence of mercury [13, 14], which was used to treat syphilis in his era. Congenital syphilis is also not a valid consideration, because even though Beethoven's father was an alcoholic, there is no evidence that he was sexually promiscuous. Beethoven also lacked any of the accompanying features of congenital syphilis such as skin rash, nasal discharge, ulcers of the nose and palate, bony deformities, corneal scarring, or dental abnormalities.

3.6 Lead poisoning

Lead poisoning has been previously considered to be the cause of Beethoven's hearing loss, but has been dismissed because he lacked wrist drop, or weakness of the extensor muscles that elevate the wrist. This is invariably present with classic lead poisoning. This classic lead toxicity, however, usually occurs with exposure to high lead levels over a few years' time. Those with low-level exposure over a longer time have mood disturbances, abnormal liver and kidney function, gastrointestinal disturbances, and pain and tingling in the hands and feet. Elevated levels of lead were found in Beethoven's hair (see **Figure 1**) and deep in the bone, consistent with exposure over a long period of time [13, 14]. This constellation of symptoms was described in a group of 151 patients in Latvia [15] and was similar to those experienced by Beethoven. It is important to note that a black lead line on gingival tissues, seen with classic lead poisoning, nor disturbance in the sense of taste, was reported neither in these patients nor by Beethoven.

3.7 The sense of taste

One of the amazing functions of the pharynx is the sense of taste. Taste buds for sweet, sour, bitter, and salt are found in the oral cavity and the or-pharynx, and even

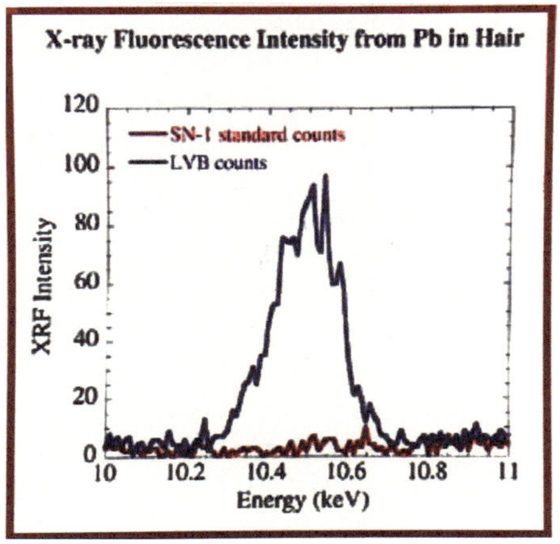

Figure 1.
X-ray fluorescence intensity levels in Beethoven's hair compared with normal levels.

in the hypopharynx. The sensation of taste or gustatory sensation is transmitted by way of both the lingual nerve *via* the seventh cranial nerve, and the pharyngeal, or ninth carnival nerve. The sense of smell is integrally involved with the sense of taste in that part of tasting foods is smelling them. Therefore, a loss of the sense of smell will make food taste bland. This has been very prevalent during the pandemic and can cause temporary as well as persistent loss. Taste disturbance is most commonly a side effect of medicine that often produces a metallic taste in the mouth. It can also be caused by viral illnesses, head injury, oral hygiene problems, tonsillectomy, stroke, and heavy metals such as lead.

3.8 Gastrointestinal problems

A recent article discusses the many medical symptoms Beethoven had during his life [16]. Although lead can account for several symptoms, such as abdominal pain or colic, it is also possible that he had irritable bowel syndrome to explain his gastrointestinal problems, and the pain in his hands and feet could have represented a rheumatological syndrome. Cirrhosis and chronic pancreatitis seen at death were attributable to his alcohol consumption, but lead could also have contributed to the cirrhosis. His kidney damage could have been caused by lead, but also by pyelonephritis.

3.9 Paget's disease

The provocative article written in 2017 mentioned in the introduction [5] deserves close scrutiny as it is well written by Oiseth, a pathologist. He disagrees with the original finding of prior pathologists [4]. There appear to be a number of flaws with his approach, which is largely based on the findings of a thickened skull on gross examination at the autopsy, which is consistent with Paget's disease. However, as he himself wrote, there are other causes of a thickened skull. One of these is hyperparathyroidism which the author suggests he had due to chronic renal disease. A gross examination is the initial examination to draw up a differential diagnosis, and then, the microscopic examination is used to confirm the diagnosis. The prior pathologists did a microscopic exam and found no evidence of Paget's disease. Oiseth dismisses this with the fact that Paget's disease of the skull is not uniform and may undergo remodeling, so normal bone may be seen in the final phase of the disease. This is something those who did the original exam were well aware of, but perhaps they did get a sample that lacked microscopic evidence of Paget's disease. This seems extremely unlikely, as they examined three large pieces of bone from the parietal and occipital areas of the skull. However, Oiseth fails to point out that a gross exam was also done on the middle ear, which was found to be normal. It would seem likely that microscopic fractures, fixation of the stapes footplate, or fissures of the otic capsule would have been seen as sequelae of the active process, since the hearing loss that is associated with Paget's usually involves the middle ear. It is also likely that an irregular surface of the temporal bone would have been noted from prior active disease.

Oiseth admits that lead poisoning cannot be dismissed entirely, but then makes the same error as other authors that have dismissed lead poisoning, by noting the lack of other neurologic manifestations. Although the article in The Laryngoscope was cited by him [4], he apparently read only the title and did not even read the abstract that states that chronic low-level lead exposure like Beethoven had does not result in motor deficits that are usually seen with acute lead poisoning. This also explains why the acoustic nerve, a sensory nerve, was shrunken with lead damage, but the facial nerve, a motor nerve, was left untouched. Beethoven's loss started in his twenties, whereas only 3% of patients with Paget's disease are under 40.

He also mentions that Beethoven had recruitment, which is an abnormal sensitivity to loud sounds, due to impingement of Paget's disease on the cochlear nerve as evidence of a sensorineural loss and not of otosclerosis. By this, he demonstrates his lack of understanding of the term sensorineural, which is an inclusive term comprising a loss from either the nerve, the cochlea, or both. Patients with hearing loss from the cochlear nerve do not have recruitment, as this is a symptom of disease in the cochlea itself. Again this underlies the difficulty of someone not familiar with hearing loss to conjecture as to its causes. Recruitment is fully discussed in the article in The Laryngoscope [7]. Therefore, it is very unlikely that Paget's disease caused Beethoven's hearing loss.

3.10 Where did the lead come from?

Although lead can come from a variety of sources such as dishes, lead-lined wine flasks, lead crystal, or mineral water at spas, Beethoven's expenditures for wine were excessive [17]. He drank wine at every meal. Although Beethoven's personal secretary never mentioned that he had a problem with alcohol, his physicians were well aware of it. His secretary did say that "Beethoven preferred wine of the heights around buda to every other" [18]. Lead was added to this inexpensive wine to improve the flavor. In addition to his father, Beethoven's family had a history of alcohol abuse. It is interesting that George Frederic Handel also had lead poisoning [19].

3.11 Recent additional evidence

A fascinating patient in Italy was reported in 2021 that dramatically emphasized the relationship that lead has to Beethoven's deafness [20]. A 64-year-old woman presented with a slowly progressive hearing loss. She also complained of abdominal pain and tingling in her upper extremities like Beethoven. An audiogram showed a moderately severe hearing loss. Elevated levels of lead were found in her blood and urine. An examination of possible lead sources revealed that she used a cooking pan with a worn ceramic surface that released lead into her food. She underwent chelation with ethylenediaminetetraacetic acid disodium salt which was injected into her to bind to the lead and allow it to be excreted from the body. After 1 year, her symptoms had all resolved, and her hearing was stabilized.

3.12 How did hearing loss affect Beethoven as a person?

Hearing loss can be very debilitating. This was especially true with Beethoven whose livelihood was dependent on his hearing. His loss caused him to be depressed, and at one time, the depression became so severe that he considered taking his own life [8]. Poignant is the picture of him when his ninth symphony was first performed. He was the honorary conductor and faced the orchestra. When the performance was finished, the contralto soloist had to turn him around to face the audience in order for him to see their applause, as he could not hear it [21]. It also significantly influenced his relationships with others. He was largely a solitary figure. He would very much have liked to have been married, but women generally found him eccentric. One cannot comprehend the depth of sorrow that this disability engendered in this gifted man.

3.13 How did his hearing loss affect his ability to compose?

On long walks that he liked to take, he would hear music in his head and write it down on a sketch pad. He did not just hear the melody, and later harmonize the parts, he heard it in its entirety [22]. With his loss of hearing, he was not able to check his music on the piano, but his superb ability to hear intervals in his head left his ability to compose unaffected. His music has been held in high esteem for over two centuries and continues to inspire millions. He recognized the great gift that he had to give to mankind and was consummately successful in doing so. Although Beethoven's hearing loss did not affect the quality of his music, his Eroica and 5th Symphony, the opera Fidelio, and the Egmont and Coriolan overtures reflect his heroic resolve and determination to conquer his suicidal thoughts and go on creating [23]. This heroic attitude is also heard in the Waldstein and Appassionata Sonatas, three string quartets opus 59, and the oratorio Christ on the Mount of Olives.

4. Conclusion

The best current evidence is that the most likely cause of Beethoven's hearing loss was his consumption of wine tainted with lead. Fortunately, it did not affect his ability to compose.

Author details

Michael Stevens
University of Utah School of Medicine, Salt Lake City, Utah, USA

*Address all correspondence to: 8.michael.stevens.6@gmail.com

References

[1] Goss C, editor. Anatomy of the Human Body. 27th ed. Philadelphia: Lea and Febiger; 1961. p. 1135

[2] Tarabichi M, Naimi M. Transtympanic dilation of the eustachian tube during chronic ear surgery. Acta Otolaryngologica. 2018;**135**:640-644. DOI: 10.3109/00016489.2015.1009640

[3] Poe D et al. Balloon dilation of the eustachian tube for dilatory dysfunction. A randomized controlled trial. The Laryngoscope. 2018;**128**:1200-1206. DOI: 10.1002/lary.26827

[4] Jessere H, Bankl H. Was Beethoven's deafness caused by Paget's Disease? Report of findings and study of skull fragments of Ludwig van Beethoven. Laryngology Rhinology Otology. 1966;**65**:592-597

[5] Oiseth SJ. Beethoven's autopsy revisited: A pathologist sounds a final note. Journal of Medical Biology. 2017;**25**:135-147. DOI: 10.1177/0967772015575803

[6] Sonnergaard JM. Ockham's razor applied on pharmaceutical powder compaction models. Journal of Pharmaceutical Sciences. 2021:110;989-996

[7] Stevens MH, Jacobsen T, Crofts AK. Lead and the deafness of Ludwig van Beethoven. The Laryngoscope. 2013;**123**:2854-2858. DOI: 10.1002/lary.24120

[8] Anderson E. The Letters of Beethoven. Vol. 1. New York, N.Y: St. Martin's Press; 1961. p. 60

[9] Shearer PD. The deafness of Beethoven: An audiologic and Medical overview. American Journal of Otology. 1990;**11**:1-5

[10] Karmody CS, Bachor ES. The deafness of Ludwig van Beethoven: An immunopathy. Otology Neurotology. 2005;**26**:809-814. DOI: 10.1097/01.mao.0000178149.36881.14

[11] Davies PJ. Ludwig van Beethoven: An autoimmune deafness? History of the Science of Medicine. 1995;**29**:271-276

[12] McCabe BF. The deafness of Beethoven. Annals of Otology Rhinology and Laryngology. 2004;**113**:585-589. DOI: 10.1177/000318940411300702

[13] US Department of Energy News Release of the Argonne National laboratory. Research Proves Beethoven Suffered from Lead Poisoning. October 17, 2000.

[14] US Department of Energy News Release of the Argonne National laboratory. Researchers Confirm Lead as cause of Beethoven's Illness. December 6, 2005.

[15] Reubens O, Logina I, Kravale I, Eglite M, Donaghy M. Peripheral neuropathy in chronic occupational inorganic lead exposure: Clinical and electrophysiological study. Journal of Neurology Neurosurgery and Psychiatry. 2001;**71**:200-204

[16] Fellin R, Reichert J. Haven't I always been a sickly person? Controversies about L. van Beethoven's illnesses. European Journal of Internal Medicine. 2020;**78**:47-48. DOI: 10.1016/j.ejim.2020.04.001

[17] Forbes E, editor. Life of Beethoven. Princeton, NJ: Princeton University Press; 1967. p. 135

[18] McArdle D. Beethoven as I Knew Him. New York, NY: Dover; 1996. p. 349

[19] Hunter D. Miraculous recovery? Handel's illnesses, the narrative tradition of heroic strength, and the oratorio turn. Eighteenth Century Music. 2006;**3**: 253-267. DOI: 10.1002/lary.28464

[20] Brotto D, Fellin R, Sorrentino F, Gheller F, Trevisi P, Bovo R. A modern case sheds light on a classical Enigma: Beethoven's deafness. The Laryngoscope. 2021;**131**:129-185

[21] Davies PJ. Beethoven in Person, His Deafness, Illnesses, and Death. Westport, CT: Greenwood Press; 2001

[22] Harrison P. The effect of deafness on musical composition. Journal of the Royal Society of Medicine. 1988;**81**:598

[23] Carner M. Beethoven's Deafness and the Heroic Element in His Music. Bericht uber den internationalen musiksenschaft Kongress. Bonn; n.p. 1970. p. 360

Section 2

The Incredible Structure and Function

Chapter 3

Esophagus

Suhaib A.H. AL-Taai

Abstract

The manuscript aims to include gross anatomical and histological structure of the esophagus. The esophagus is one of the important portions of the digestive system. Definition of the esophagus is, a muscular tube which is extended from the pharynx floor until the stomach. Its function is to transport the food particles from the oro-pharynx by swallowing operation on way esophageal opening during pharynx to the stomach. Morphology, the esophagus is a long cylindrical structure, which is divided into three segments, the upper portion is called cervical, either intermediate is the thoracic part, and the lower segment is named abdominal, which is attached with the stomach. Muscles of the esophagus are skeletal or striated muscles in the upper segment toward the pharynx, striated and smooth in the middle, either latest segment of the esophagus consists of smooth muscles only. The esophageal structure is different from other types of animals. These differences depend on the nature of food consumption. Histology, the esophagus contains four layers called tunics. First tunics is called the mucosa (epithelia have stratified squamous non-keratin, lamina properia, and muscularis), the next tunics is sub mucosa (connective tissue) with spread to find esophageal glands, either the other two layers are tunica muscularis (outer layer included longitudinal orientation and inner muscles is circular orientations), circular muscle orientation is not clearly circular in each part of the esophagus, but these fibers become more actually at lower parts of the esophagus. Either the muscularis and adventitia (loose connective tissue) without being covered by mesothelium.

Keywords: esophagus, anatomy, histology

1. Introduction

The digestive system is one of important systems, that sustains digest and absorbs nutritional materials and expels as feces the remaining waste. The digestive system includes the mouth cavity, pharynx, esophagus, stomach, small, and large intestine until anus [1, 2].

The esophagus in gray mongoose is a narrow musculo–membranous folded tube extending from the oropharynx to the stomach. The esophagus is ventrally bordered by the trachea, dorsally by the vertebral column, and laterally by the carotid artery; a similar location is also observed in canine [3].

As in domestic animals [4, 5], the esophagus of gray mongoose is divided into three parts, cervical, thoracic, and abdominal.

The cervical region of the esophagus passed dorsally to the trachea but turns to the left side of the trachea before entering the thoracic cavity. The course of the esophagus is akin to that of a canine [6]. Meanwhile, it appeared to deviate slightly to the left in the cervical region only and runs along the dorsal aspect of the trachea in the laboratory rat [7].

So, the abdominal portion of the esophagus in gray mongoose is short, 1 cm in length, and expanded to the stomach till the end, while in cat, the length of the caudal part of the esophagus is 3 cm. However, these variations may be due to individual's factors such as height, body weight, and gender [8].

The internal wall of the mongoose esophagus showed longitudinal folds all over its length, this may be given more capacity for a large mass of food to pass through, taking into consideration that the gray mongoose is voracious and eat food quickly. Whereas in cats, the presence of transverse folds is only restricted in distal thirds of the thoracic esophagus [8]. And this phenomenon in humans has been termed a feline esophagus (**Figure 1**) [9].

1.1 Cranial gastrointestinal tract

The cranial gastrointestinal tract involves the mouth cavity, pharynx, esophagus, stomach, and duodenum. This outlines the embryonic boundaries between foregut and midgut and is also the division that clinicians commonly used to describe gastro-intestinal bleeding as either cranial or caudal in origin. The duodenum may seem to be a unified organ when dissected, but it is divided into four segments based on role, position, and interior anatomy, descending, horizontal, and ascending [1].

1.2 Gross Anatomy of the esophagus

Anatomical differences in the esophagus between species reflect modification to different foods consumed by different species and behavioral adaptations [10]. The esophagus 'gross anatomy has been described previously, have three regions; cervical, thoracic, and abdominal [5] in the dog.

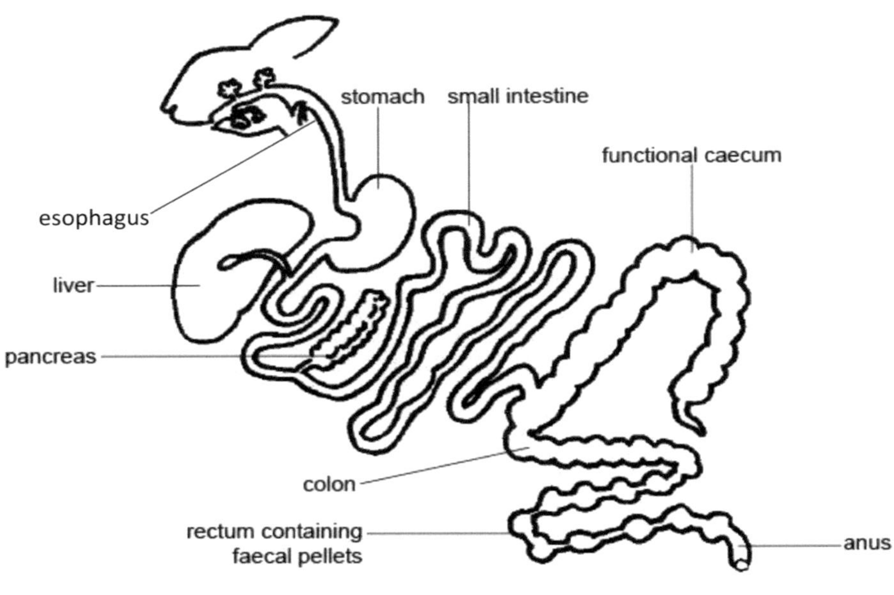

Figure 1.
Parts of the digestive system in rabbit.

The esophagus is a cylinder structure that often prolongs from the pharynx to the cardiac opening of the stomach, the length of the esophagus as measured in 8–13 cm adult cats varied between 17.5–21 cm. The esophagus would have been about 30 cm long in dogs and about 2 cm in diameter [11].

The esophagus of the goat was 45–50 cm long; the esophagus of the cervical part was 13–15 cm long. On the other hand, in bovine, the esophagus length was 90–105 cm long [12]. The length of the esophagus in sheep is 45 cm long and the diameter in the pharynx was 1.8 and 2.5 cm in the cardia. The length of the esophagus in the horse is 125–150 cm [12]. The cervical part is 75 cm [13, 14]. The camel esophagus is an elongated tube structure of large capacity; it can be 1–2 m long [14].

The bovine esophagus length is 90–105 cm, the cervical region is 42–49 cm. Measurements of the esophagus diameter are unreliable due to its dilatability in the living animal. The esophagus in sheep is 45 cm in length, 12 increases in diameter from 1.8 cm in the pharynx to 2.5 cm in the stomach junction [8]. In canine, the cervical portion of the esophagus dorsally to the trachea but turns in the middle of the neck to the left and continues through the thoracic inlet to this direction. The esophagus collapses in its latent state and can distend to accommodate fluid and solid material. The esophagus begins at the inferior margin of the cricopharyngeus muscle and extends to the lower esophageal sphincter [15].

Topographically, in cats, the esophagus starts from the pharynx and extends through the length of the cervical area on the dorsal side of the trachea; it remains completely straight on the dorsal surface of the trachea between the 1st and 7th cervical vertebrae. Cervical esophagus length is about 4 cm; it is about 30 percent of the length of the body [16, 17]. However, the first part of the esophagus in canine and other domestic animals is located dorsally to trachea but turned left in the middle of the neck, retaining this position through the thoracic outline [17].

In guinea pig, the cervical part of the esophagus deviates slightly to the left only in the cervical region, the dorsal aspect of the trachea follows mostly mid sagittal. Its length is approximately 30 mm, the diameter is approximately 2 mm (Langer, 2002). In the rat, only in the cervical region, the esophagus slightly deviates to the left and passes midsagittally along the trachea's dorsal aspect with a total length of 7.5 cm [6].

The esophagus in rabbits is accompanied laterally by vagosympathetic trunk and carotid artery along the cervical course. It lies dorsally to the trachea and ventrally to the cervical muscles, prolonging from the pharynx to the thoracic outline, approximately 7 cm long [18].

The gross investigation of the llama esophagus shows the cervical part placed dorsally and on the left side of the trachea. The total length is about 121 cm, the cervical portion is about 80 cm long [19].

The cat's thoracic esophagus is located adjacent to essential structures, such as the trachea, vertebrae, lungs, heart, blood vessels, and lymphatics. The cranial third of the thoracic esophagus seems to have an intimate relationship with the trachea; the caudal third has quite an intimate relationship with the aorta [7].

Topographic morphology of thoracic esophagus in dogs made an appearance within the mediastinum left to the trachea, continuously differentiating dorsal to trachea between both the left sub clavian artery and the left lung in the peri-cardiac mediastinum. At the level of the 2nd thoracic vertebra between both the left aortic arch and the right azygous vein, the esophagus reaches the base of the heart dorsal to the trachea and the left bronchus. It passes at the level of the 5th rib above the tracheal bifurcation and passes between the caudal lung lobes toward the esophageal hiatus at the level of the 10th thoracic vertebra [20].

The thoracic segment in the feline extends from the thoracic inlet, where it is located to the left of the trachea, passes through the bifurcation of the trachea, and reaches caudally to the esophageal hiatus of the diaphragm [21].

In laboratory animals, the thoracic portion course began as shown at the level of the 1st rib, at the thoracic inlet; its dorsal situation to the trachea has still been maintained. It is positioned between the lung lobes at both the tracheal bifurcation and passes over the base of the heart. After its origin, the thoracic aorta passes obliquely to its left over the esophagus. The thoracic part was approximately 20 mm long [22].

In the rabbits, the esophagus at the thoracic outline has remained dorsal to the trachea and continues as the thoracic esophagus until the bifurcation between the lung lobes of the trachea [23].

The esophagus is enacted through the dorsal thoracic inlet to the trachea. Throughout the mediastinum, in adult lamas, the thoracic esophagus reached to the right of the aortic arch dorsal to the heart base [19].

The abdominal esophagus stretches from those in the diaphragm hiatus to that of the sphincter of the stomach's cardia, about 1 cm long, the base of the esophagus progressions smoothly into the stomach's cardiac orifice. The abdominal portion of either the esophagus is situated on the dorsal border to that of the left liver lobe in the esophageal impression. Lower esophageal sphincter muscles at either the ends of the esophagus, but there is no clear anatomical demarcation of the limits of the sphincters [24].

In the cat, the abdominal esophagus is short, expanded, enters its abdomen from the esophageal hiatus with either the vagus trunk, commonly 3 cm or less in length, and binds to either the gastroesophageal junction [17]

In the dog, the abdominal section of either the esophagus is wedge-shaped. Dorsally, the esophagus joins the stomach and sits ventrally on the notches at both the thin dorsal border of the liver's caudate lobe [11, 21].

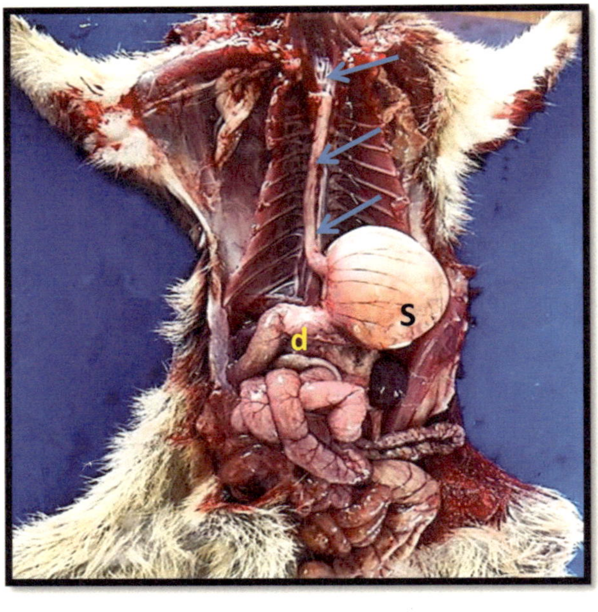

Figure 2.
Ventral view of squirrel shows cervical, thoracic, and abdominal esophagus (blue arrow), stomach (S), duodenum(d) [30].

The abdominal part, that same esophagus in the laboratory mouse is short (several mm length) easily noticed [25].

As the esophagus passed through a slit-like esophageal hiatus in the cat, the surrounding muscle of the right diaphragmatic crus, as in man and dog, supports it [26].

In cattle, the caudal end of the esophagus is usually slit-like about 2–3 cm, [27, 28].

In rabbits, the esophagus passes in the abdominal cavity through esophageal hiatus ventral to the thoracic aorta and continues as a short abdominal course of about 1 cm connected with the stomach at lesser curvature [29].

The abdominal portion of the esophagus in llama was very short, approximately 2 cm in length. Esophageal outer diameter began gradually enlarged [29].

Internally, in feline the transverse folds is only present, whilst another study found longitudinal folds in the cranial and middle parts of the cervical esophageal walls and transverse folds in the caudal part [29].

In the cat, internal appearance shows that the caudal portion of the esophagus has transverse folds [30].

In squirrels, the esophagus is featured muscular tubular like, it's located at beginning of oropharynx to stomach. It is divided into three parts, 1st cervical and 2nd segments are thoracic and abdominal segments. In this paragraph, the study shows esophagus of squirrels is extended from and endpoints corresponded between the 6th cervical vertebra and 11th thoracic ribs (**Figure 2**) [30].

1.3 Histological structure of esophagus

The histological findings of the esophagus consist of muscular tubes, which is star-like lumen, filled with or without desquamating cells. The structure of the esophagus includes the 4th tunicus (mucosa, submucosa, muscularis, and adventitia). We observed the epithelia, stratified squamous non-keratin. The first tuncus is called tunica mucosa has epithelia, lamina properia which includes loose connective tissue and muscular layer beneath them. The second layer is named submucosa includes connective tissue. Another consists of tunica muscularis orientation, itconsists of internal layer which is called circular muscular fibers while the outer layer is longitudinal orientation. The adventitia is the last tunica which includes loose connective tissue [30].

1.3.1 Mucosa

The tunica mucosa is divided into three portions, the first portion is called epithelium (Non-keratinized stratified squamous), which rested on the basal lamina. The second layer is lamina propia, and third layer is muscularis mucosa. Lamina propia is formed mostly of loose connective tissue in some states from collagen fibers and elastic fibers and lamina muscularis mucosa consists of some smooth muscle fibers [30].

1.3.2 Submucosa

This tunica includes dense connective tissue represented elastic and collagen fibers, irregular connective tissue. This layer consists of large blood vessels and meissner plexus, which is a group of ganglia that connects central nervous system.

1.3.3 Muscularis

Group of muscles include longitudinal and circular orientation bundles muscles form tube-like esophagus: longitudinal muscle fibers are located to inner either

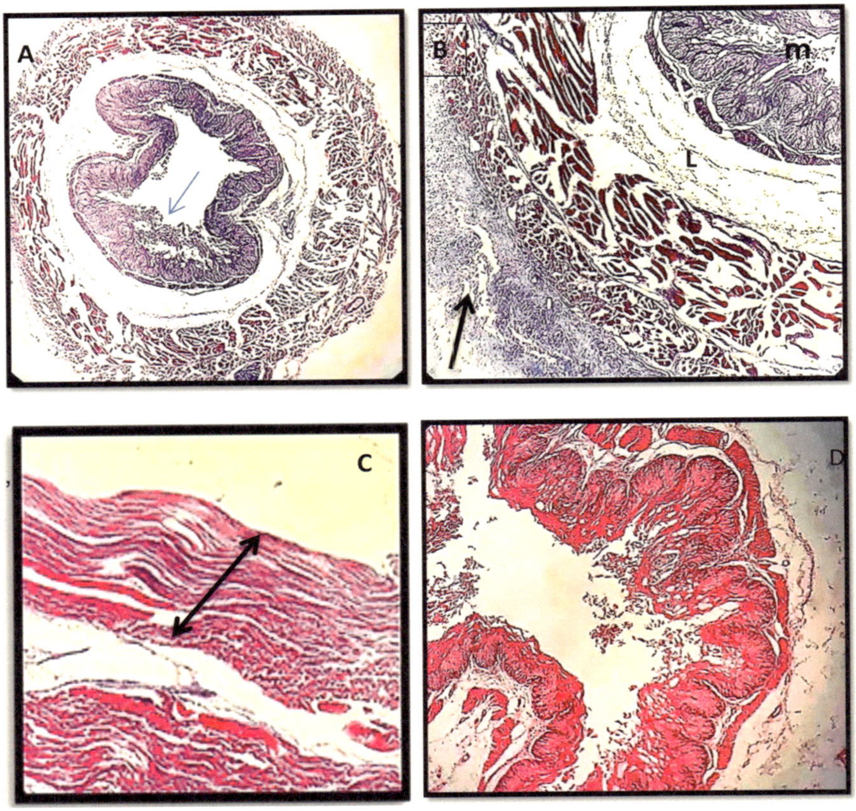

Figure 3.
Histological section of esophagus shows A, lumen contains desquamating cells (blue arrow), masson's tichome 40x. B, Mucosa (m), Loose c.t,submucosa (s), tunica adventitia (black arrow) masson's trichome 100x, C, muscularis (inner circular muscles), (IM) and (outer longitudinal muscles fibers, (OM) , H&E 100X, D, Showed mucosa and lose c.t. 100x [30].

circular muscle fibers are located externally. The muscle fibers in this portion from tunica are situated laterally within the roof of the esophagus, but these fibers extended and surround all surfaces at lower sides, and it is strongest in the lower third layer of the esophagus. Either circular muscle fibers are located under the longitudinal muscle, and the circular muscle, which is thinner to compare with longitudinal muscle. Circular muscles does not actually circular in each part of esophagus; these fibers remain most elliptic in the upper third part and become more circular at the lower third part of the esophagus. Also, these fibers do not form a regular formation but run in an irregular pattern making a shutter-like system. Spontaneous perforation of the esophagus usually occurs in the last 2 cm, and this perforation consists of the entire esophageal wall, causing mediastinitis because of gastric acid leakage. The upper part of the esophagus consists of striated muscle and the lower part consists of smooth muscle fibers [30].

1.3.4 Adventitia

This is the last layer of tunics boundary of the esophagus and is composed of loose connective tissue. Because no serosa is found on the esophagus (**Figure 3**) [30].

2. Conclusions

The esophagus is different in different kinds of animals, depending on the nature of food consumption, such aslarge animals can be contrasted with small animals e.g., squirrels, mice, rats...etc. The sphincter muscle may be missing in upper and lower parts of the esophagus in some animals, also the nature of epithelium may vary in all animals, that is, keratinize or non-keratinize, depending on the food that animals have.. Other differences are, glands of the esophagusmay be present or not in submucosa, so the distribution of desquamating cells inside the lumen. The myentric nerve plexus is very prominent in some animals and located between the outer layer of tunica muscularis and adventitia.

Author details

Suhaib A.H. AL-Taai
Veterinary Medicine College, Department of Anatomy and Histology, University of Baghdad, Baghdad, Iraq

*Address all correspondence to: dr.suhaibaltaai@gmail.com

References

[1] Jump P, Ruppert EE, Fox RS, Barnes RD. Introduction to Bilateria. In: Invertebrate Zoology. 7th ed. Devon, UK: Brooks/Cole; 2004. pp. 203-205

[2] Ruppert EE, Fox RS, Barnes RD. Introduction to Eumetazoa. In: Invertebrate Zoology. 7th ed. Devon, UK: Brooks/Cole; 2004. pp. 99-103

[3] Meyer RA, McGinley D, Posalaky Z. Effects of aspirin on tight junction structure of the canine gastric mucosa. Gastroenterology. 1986;**91**(2):351-359

[4] Stinson AW, Lois M, Calhoun ML. Textbook of Veterinary Histology (IV). Philadelphia: Lea & Febiger; 1993. pp. 153-193

[5] Evans HE and Christensen GC. Miller's anatomy of the dog. 3rd ed. Philadelphia: Saunders; 1993. pp. 501-504.

[6] Rudolf H, Stromberg MW. Digestive system. In: Anatomy of the Laboratory Rat. 1976. pp. 43-51

[7] Allouch A, Kaddi M. Surgical Anatomy of the Esophagus in Cats and Removal of Esophageal Foreign Bodies (Sneeze Spine) Using Laryngoscope Technique. 2018

[8] Noh HM, Fishman EK, Forastiere AA, Bliss DF, Calhoun PS. CT of the esophagus: Spectrum of disease with emphasis on esophageal carcinoma. Radiographics. 1995;**15**(5):1113-1134

[9] David A, Soybel W. Oxford Textbook of Medicine: Sections 18-33. Oxford, UK: Oxford University Press; 2005. p. 511

[10] Furth EE, Rubesin SE and Rose D. Radiologic-Pathologic Conferences of the Hospital of the University of Pennsylvania, Feline Esophagus. 2017

[11] Bello A, Onyeanusi BI, Sonfada ML, Adeyanju JB, Umaru MA, Onu JE. Gross embryonic diffrentiation of the stomach of the one humped camel (camelus dromedarius). Anatomy & Physiology: Current Research. 2014;**4**:1

[12] Miller ME. The digestive system and abdomen. Pancreas. In: Miller ME, editor. Anatomy of the Dog. Philadelphia: W. B. Saunders Company; 1964. pp. 706-710

[13] Getty R, Sisson S. Sisson and Grossman's the Anatomy of the Domestic Animals (No. DEPOSITO FV). 1975

[14] Ghoshal NG, Bal HS. Comparative morphology of the stomach of some laboratory mammals. Laboratory Animals. 1998;**23**(1):21-29

[15] Nickel R, Schumnier A, Seiferle E. Lehrbuch der Anatomie der Haustiere. In: Habermehl K-H, Vollmerhaus B, Wilkens H, editors. Eingeweide. Vol. 2. Berlin: Blackwell; 1995. pp. 144-147

[16] Dyce KM, Sack WO, Wensing CJG. Textbook of Veterinary Anatomy. 4th ed. London: Saunders an imprint of Elsevier Inc.; 2010

[17] Long JD, Orlando RC. Anatomy, histology, embryology, and developmental abnormalities of the esophagus. In: Feldman M, Fieldman LS, Sleisenger MH, editors. Gastrointestinal and Liver Diseases. Philadelphia: WB Saunders; 2002. pp. 551-560

[18] Deprem T, Taşçi SK, Bingöl SA, Sari EK, Aslan Ş, Ilhan S. Histological and histochemical studies on the structure of pancreatic Histological and

histochemical studies on the structure of pancreatic ducts of the goose (Anser anser). Turkish Journal of Veterinary and Animal Sciences. 2015;**39**(1):62-68

[19] Sukon P, Timm KI, Valentine BA. Esophageal Anatomy of the Llama (Lama glama). International Journal of Morphology. 2009;**27**(3)

[20] Alsafy MA, El-Gendy SA. Gastroesophageal junction of Anatolian shepherd dog: A study by topographic anatomy, scanning electron and light microscopy. Veterinary Research Communications. 2012;**36**:63-69

[21] Sivarao DV, Goyal RK. Functional anatomy and physiology of the upper esophageal sphincter. The American Journal of Medicine. 2000;**108**(4):27-37

[22] Das P, Ranjan R. Gross Morphology and Histo-Architecture of Rabbit Esophagus. department of. Veterinary Anatomy and Histology, West Bengal University of Animal and Fishery Sciences. 2016;**93**(05):40-44

[23] Tamate H, Yamada, j. Histological and immunocytochemical observation of hindstomach of the collared peccary (Dicotylestayacu). The Japanese Journal of veterinary Science. 1983;**45**(5): 547-549

[24] Goyal RK, Sivarao DV. Functional anatomy and physiology of swallowing and esophageal motility. In: Catell OD, Richter JE, editors. The Esophagus. 3rd ed. Philadelphia: Lippincott Williams & Wilkins; 1993. p. 23

[25] Berghes C, Tanase P, Parvu M, Dinu C, Cuca D. Contributions to the study of the esophagus and stomach morphology in guinea pig. Scientific Papers Animal Science and Biotechnologies. 2011;**44**(2):150-154

[26] Cedric G, Jerry FSF, Henry E. Studies of the gastroesophageal sphincter mechanism: The role of the phrenoesophageal membrane. Surgary. 1970;**67**:735-740

[27] Habel RE. Guide to the Dissection of Domestic Ruminants. Ann Arbor, MI: Edwards Bro. Inc.; 1964

[28] Church DC. Digestive physiology and nutrition of ruminants. In: Digestive Physiology. 2nd ed. Vol. 1. Corvallis, OR: O&B Books, Inc.; 1979

[29] Ranjan R, Das P. Gross morphology and histo-architecture of rabbit esophagus. Department of veterinary anatomy and histology, West Bengal University of Animal and Fishery Sciences, Kolkata-700 037. Indian Veterinary Journal. 2016;**93**(5):40-44

[30] AL-Taai SAH, Nsaif RH, Almayahi MS. Histomorphological study of esophagus in squirrel (Sciurus anomalus). Biochemical and Cellular Archives. 2021;**21**:1391-1394

Chapter 4

Adenoids: Their Importance and the Role of Preserving Adenoids When Planning for Adenotonsillectomy

Subramaniam Vinayak and Mohak Kumar

Abstract

Adenoid is a secondary lymphoid organ located in the nasopharynx. Its location plays an important role in the host defence of the upper respiratory tract. Adenoid hypertrophy is common in children of age 8–15 which cause symptoms ranging from mouth breathing, hyponasal speech, snoring, obstructive sleep apnoea long term sequelae of which could be neurocognitive abnormalities like learning difficulties and below-average intelligent quotient (adenoid facies----idiotic look), and a higher risk of cardiovascular morbidity(e.g.: decreased right ventricular ejection fraction, left ventricular hypertrophy). To name a few more patients with adenoid hypertrophy are more susceptible to get symptoms suggestive of chronic sinusitis, recurrent otitis media. Tonsils and Adenoids are usually larger in children but the trend to shrink as age progresses, making it all the more a reason to be conservative in the management of treating adenoid hypertrophy by employing corticosteroid nasal sprays.

Keywords: adenoid hypertrophy, adenoidectomy, adenotonsillectomy

1. Introduction

The Adenoid and Tonsils are lumps of tissue and they are considered as lymphoid organs which play a vital role in a person's immunity.

Immunoglobulin G3, and AI antibodies are prevalent antibodies in the adenoid tissue [1].

Adenotonsillectomy in the case of adenotonsillar hypertrophy is the typical management strategy but with potential surgical complications have prompted to think of non-surgical alternatives [2], and moreover a connection between allergy and adenoid hypertrophy made to think of using intranasal corticosteroid sprays as an alternative to the surgical option and thus preserve the adenoid tissue.

2. History

Meyer [3] first described this mucosa-associated lymphatic tissue in 1868.

3. Embryology

The Adenoid tissue develops from the subepithelial infiltrations of lymphocytes after the 16th week of embryonic life, the enlargement of this lymphatic tissue begins and continues until age 5 to 7 [3], the fusion of two lateral primordia the neurocranium [3] and viscerocranium leads to the formation of the adenoid tissue.

4. Anatomy

The Adenoid tissue is a mass of lymphatic tissue situated in the roof of the nasopharynx behind the nasal cavity. It is a midline structure.

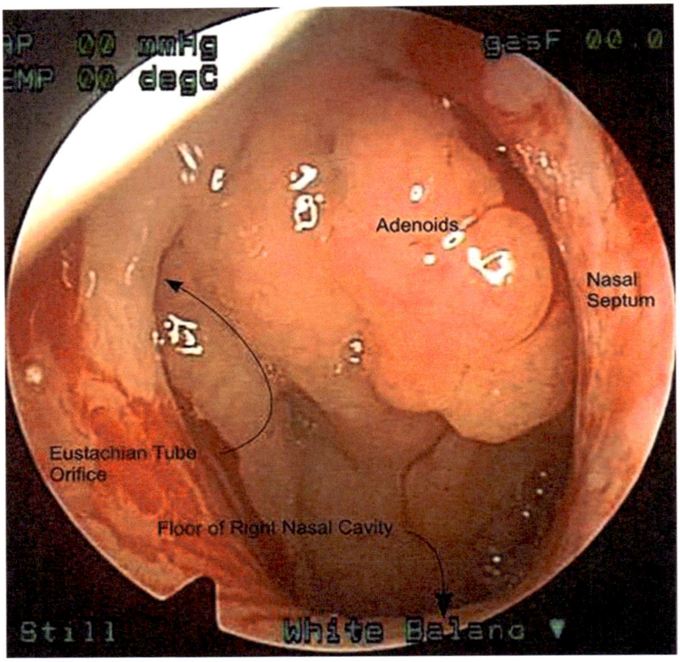

Endoscopic picture of adenoid tissue.

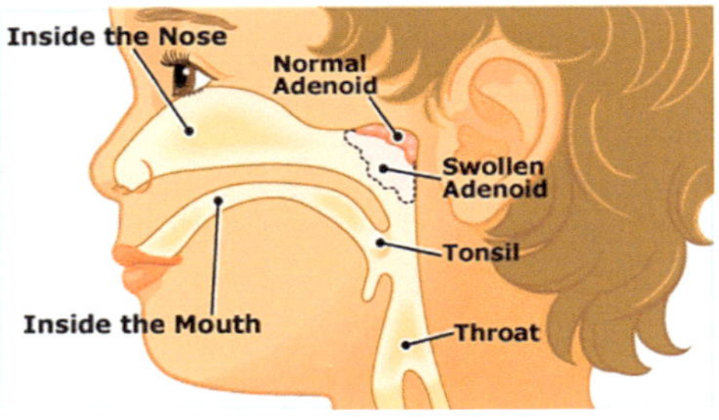

Picture showing the position of the adenoid and tonsil.

It is pyramidal in shape [3].

It forms a part of the Waldeyer's ring which comprises of 1) palatine tonsil, 2) lingual tonsil, and the 3) tubal tonsil. It is also called Pharyngeal Tonsil/Nasopharyngeal Tonsil.

The arterial supply [3] is from the basisphenoid artery,

ascending pharyngeal artery,

ascending palatine artery,

pharyngeal branch of the maxillary artery,

tonsillar branch of the facial artery,

and the artery of the pterygoid canal, as regards the venous drainage is the pharyngeal plexus which eventually drains into the facial veins and internal jugular veins.

The lymphatic drainage comprises the pharyngomaxillary space and retropharyngeal lymph nodes.

The nerve supply being is mainly the pharyngeal plexus,

which contains fibres of the cranial nerves 9th,10th,11th. The main nerve supply originates from the 9th, and 10th.

5. Histology

Adenoid tissue is divided into four lobes with seromucinous glands which is interposed within the tissue. It is composed of respiratory epithelium.

6. Physiology

Adenoid tissue along with the other structures that form the Waldyeres ring are the first line of defence against ingested or inhaled pathogens. The tissues of the ring are involved in the development of the T cells and B cells.

On the surface are specialised antigen capture cells (ACC), M cells,which uptake the pathogenic antigens and then alert the B cells [3] this proliferates in the germinal layers which produce IgA Immunoglobulins, thus helping in the developing an immunologic memory.

7. Discussion

Putting the above details into perspective the idea of doing an adenoidectomy as a routine when we otorhinolaryngologists plan to an adenotonsillectomy should be given a serious thought, unless and until the patients suffer's from obstructive symptoms, or repeated attacks of Acute Otitis Media as an adjuvant to Gromett insertion.

Thus, this chapter is an attempt to drive home the point using a study [4] that I have done and the same has been published in a reputed journal, the details of which could be got in the references which are at the end of the chapter.

This study was conducted in a Government Hospital in India in a place called Sirsi, Karnataka.

This study comprised of selecting patients of the age group 5–15 yrs. as this is the most common age group of presentation.

The result of this study suggested that when a patient with the presentation of only symptoms of enlarged adenoids along with chronic tonsillitis and no other added symptoms like those suggestive of Acute Otitis Media one need not think of doing adenotonsillectomy as usually done but instead we should think of the conservative mode of treatment in terms of using steroidal nasal sprays which have been proven to regress the size of the adenoid tissue.

Secondly, the adenoid tissue as earlier mentioned due to its location (a so-called blind spot) could cause problems in case of a bleed and due to its proximity to important structures like the all-important Eustachian Tube could cause damage or scarring to the orifice in turn leading to long term complications, at times after surgery one could leave some amount of tissue if large adenoids which could lead to persisting complains, and moreover the adenoid tissue tend to regress most of the times as one's age progresses and in the long run helping the individual with his or her immunity status(as mentioned earlier) thus giving time its due and being conservative [5] we could land up saving adenoids more often than not.

8. Conclusion or take home message

1. Drawing lines of similarity between conserving the nature at times of global warming and doing conservative surgeries like FESS, one could add this concept too, i.e.: avoidance of doing Adenoidectomy as routine in doing an Adenotonsillectomy.

2. As discussed earlier the Adenoids play an important part in maintaining the individual's immune status and moreover the Adenoids regress as age progress it is better that one preserves the Adenoids.

3. Due to the location of the adenoid tissue and its intricate blood supply it could cause complications like bleeding which could be difficult to localise and stop, and there could be scarring of the Eustachian tube orifice which could lead to complications involving the maintaining of middle ear pressure and related issues.

4. At times one could leave behind some of the adenoid tissue and this could lead to symptoms of adenoid hypertrophy resurfacing.

5. One would be justified in doing Adenoidectomy only when the patient presents with associated complications of Adenoid hypertrophy like (a) Sleep Apnoea Syndrome, (b) Recurrent attacks of Acute Suppurative Otitis Media.

6. Administration of Fluticasone Nasal Sprays [5] in monthly tapered dose has shown promising results in the regression of the size of the Adenoid tissue and thus reducing symptoms like mouth breathing and snoring.

Thus, putting all the above points into consideration, it would be apt to say that one should give this sort of conservative form of treatment a serious thought and try saving the all-important ADENOID tissue.

Author details

Subramaniam Vinayak[1*] and Mohak Kumar[2]

1 Pandit General Hospital, Sirsi, Karnataka, India

2 DY Patil Medical College, Pune, Maharashtra, India

*Address all correspondence to: vinoo121071@gmail.com

References

[1] Turkoglu Babakurban S, Aydm E. Adenoidectomy: current approaches and review of the literature. Kulak Burun Bogaz Ithis Derg. 2016;**26**(3):181-190

[2] Scadding G. Non–Surgical treatment of adenoidal hypertrophy: the role of treating IgE mediated inflammation. Pediatric Allergy and Immunology. 2010;**21**(8):1095-1106

[3] Anatomy, Head and Neck, Adenoids Ani Mnatsakanian; Jenna R. Heil; Sandeep Sharma. Available from: http://www.ncbi.nih.gov/books/NBK538137

[4] Vinayak SE. Role of Adenoidectomy in Adenotonsillectomy: An Observational Study. Clinical Rhinology an International Journal. 2019;**12**. DOI: 10.5005/jp-journals-10013-1360

[5] Kuyucu S, Kuyucu N, Unal S, Apaydin D. Nonsurgical treatment of adenoidal hypertrophy with cefuroxime axetil and intranasal mometasone furoate combination. Journal of Pediatric Infection. 2007;**1**:6-12

Section 3

The Incredible Resection and Reconstruction on Pharyngeal Cancer

Chapter 5

Hypopharyngeal Cancer

Oancea Alina Lavinia Antoaneta, Berteșteanu Șerban Vifor Gabriel, Grigore Raluca and Popescu Bogdan

Abstract

Hypopharyngeal cancer is one of the most challenging pathologies regarding location, evolution, prognosis and functional implications. Since the hypopharynx is a crossroad in the digestive and respiratory pathways malignant pathology located at this site can cause dysphagia, odynophagia, respiratory distress and dysphonia. Complex anatomy and physiology of the hypopharynx make for pathology with a poor prognosis in late stages. Diagnosis and therapy are mandatory for ensuring high survival rates and as little functional impairment as possible. Therapy of hypopharyngeal cancer is a difficult test for both physician and patient. It requires a good collaboration between the ENT surgeon, pathologist, radiotherapist, chemotherapist, nutrition therapist and psychologist. Our approach to the subject is due to that data concerning this pathology is limited and the results of the overall oncology therapy are discouraging. Nonetheless, the technical steps of surgery make it difficult for ENT cancer surgeons to approach it, therefore the surgeons' experience plays a very important role in decision making and establishing a good doctor-patient relationship, both during initial therapy and follow-up. We will also present an original technique developed in our clinic for restoring the continuity of the pharynx after total circular resection using the synthetic prosthesis.

Keywords: Hypopharynx, neoplasm, pharynx reconstruction, pharynx cancer, laryngo-pharyngectomy

1. Introduction

Cancer is still a major problem of modern medicine. Research continues trying to understand the tumor biology mechanisms as well as to find new methods of effective treatment [1]. The hypopharynx is a crossroad in the upper part of the digestive and respiratory pathways and malignant appearance at this level leads to the impairment of two vital functions, breathing and feeding. It also affects speech. Therapy of this pathology creates disability for the patient under economic, social, psychological and medical aspects. Therefore, we can advocate that hypopharyngeal cancer is one of the most challenging cancers pathologies regarding location, evolution, prognosis and functional implications. Therapy of hypopharyngeal cancer is a difficult endeavor for both physician and patient and requires a multidisciplinary approach: ENT surgeon, oncologists, radiologists, vocal rehabilitation specialist, psychologist and nutritionist.

The primary purpose of the oncology management of aero-digestive malignant neoplasms is survival. Nevertheless, preserving respiratory, deglutition and speech functions are mandatory if oncology principles are not broken.

The survival rate for hypopharyngeal cancer is low despite advanced surgical techniques, radiotherapy and chemotherapy. Patients go for medical examination in advanced stages of the disease when the tumor already exceeds the mucous layer and causes cervical lymph node metastases, thus being a challenge for the medical oncology team. Hypopharyngeal cancer management requires the presence of experienced surgeons within trained oncology surgery teams due to the radical surgical therapy aimed to locally control this type of cancer. Oncology radicality overcomes the principle of function preservation which is sometimes impossible to achieve.

2. Surgical anatomy of the hypopharynx

The pharynx is a muscular-fibrous organ that belongs to the upper aero-digestive tract. It is located anteriorly to the cervical spines and posteriorly to the nasal fossae, oral cavity and larynx with which it communicates at different levels.

From a topographical perspective the pharynx is divided into 3 segments:

- superior segment – the rhinopharynx (also known as nasopharynx, epipharynx or cavum) communicates anteriorly with the nasal fossae through the two choanae.

- middle segment – the buccopharynx (also known as oropharynx or mesopharynx) communicates anteriorly with the oral cavity.

- inferior segment – the hypopharynx (also known as laryngopharynx) communicates with the larynx, extends from the upper junction with the oropharynx at the level of the hyoid bone, and is continued inferiorly with the cervical esophagus. Hypopharyngeal cancer can occur at the site of the lateral walls, piriform sinuses, posterior wall and the retro-cricoid region. The anterior wall consists of the base of the tongue, supraglottic larynx and the posterior blade of the cricoid cartilage. The lateral walls join with the outer limits of the larynx to create two grooves, the piriform sinuses, through which fluids and food pass towards the mouth of the esophagus. The hypopharynx is shaped as a three-walled pyramid (anterior, lateral, medial) with the base located up at the pharyngoepiglottic fold and the free edge of the aryepiglottic fold, and the tip located below the cricoid cartilage. The upper lateral limit of the piriform sinus is considered an oblique line on the pharyngeal lateral wall in opposition to the aryepiglottic fold. The relations of the piriform sinus with the larynx explain why malignant tumors of the hypopharynx invade the larynx early and require surgical resections by partial or total laryngectomies. The posterior wall of the hypopharynx has a close relationship with the retropharyngeal space, the prevertebral fascia, the longitudinal spinal muscles (the long muscle of the head) and has a width of 4 cm–5 cm and a height of 6 cm–7 cm. The distance between the posterior pharyngeal wall and the vertebral bodies is no greater than 1 centimeter, therefore the submucosal protrusions caused by osteophytes or by the anterior edges of the vertebral bodies can be misinterpreted as submucosal tumors. In addition, tumors of the posterior wall of the hypopharynx can invade these prevertebral soft tissues. Between the prevertebral aponeurosis and the posterior pharyngeal and esophagus wall there is a loose cellular tissue that allows surgical and approach and detachment of the two regions. From a surgical perspective, a tumor located in the retro-cricoid region that invades the upper esophageal sphincter raise special problems. Therefore, the anterior wall of the retro-cricoid region is also called "party wall". The retro-cricoid region extends from the portion immediately below the arytenoids to the upper esophageal sphincter and forms the posterior wall of the larynx in the lower region. The anatomical relations explain the extension of the tumors of the post-cricoid region to the recurrent nerve, the paratracheal lymph nodes, the thyroid gland, the common carotid artery with its terminal branches and to the vagus nerves.

From inside out, in a cross-section, the pharyngeal wall is made out of four layers: the lining mucosa represented by a multi-layered squamous cell epithelium, a fibrous stroma developed from the pharyngeal aponeurosis, the muscular layer formed by the pharynx constrictor muscles arranged circularly and the lifting muscles arranged longitudinally and the buccopharyngeal fascia located on the outside. The constrictor muscles are superior, middle and inferior. The middle and inferior constrictor muscles surround the lateral and posterior walls of the hypopharynx that continue inferiorly with the walls of the cervical esophagus. Anteriorly, the posterior cricoarytenoid muscle represents the muscular layer. Below the hyoid bone, where the middle and lower constrictor do not cross, there is a weak point of the pharyngeal lateral wall represented by the thyrohyoid membrane, which is passed through by the vessels, nerves and lymph vessels of the hypopharynx.

The pharyngo-esophageal junction, also known as "Killian's mouth of the esophagus", makes the transition between the hypopharynx and the cervical esophagus. The difficulty of diagnosing pharyngo-esophageal junction cancer is variable depending on the circumstances of appearance and development of the malignant neoplastic lesion at this site.

The branches of the external carotid artery provide the arterial supply. Venous drainage is achieved through the facial vein and pterygoid plexus to the internal jugular vein. Lymphatic circulation drains lymph from the hypopharynx to the jugular lymph nodes. The submucosal layer of the hypopharynx contains a rich lymphatic network that exits superiorly through the thyro-hyoid membrane to reach the superior and middle jugular lymph nodes and the inferior lymphatics drain into the paratracheal and middle jugular lymph nodes.

The hypopharynx is an essential organ in assuring breathing, swallowing and speech. Tumors located at this level can cause swallowing and breathing impairment, both by the mass effect (large tumors) and/or by edema caused by the lymphatic invasion. Tumor invasion of neural structures can cause pharyngeal muscle contraction impairment or intense pain with negative effects on the swallowing process and the quality of life of the patients [2].

Damage to the arytenoid cartilages or recurrent nerves by malignant neoplasia invasion can cause major respiratory impairment with tracheobronchial aspiration phenomena by paresis of the vocal cords. Peritumoral infections can cause impaired swallowing [3, 4].

3. Epidemiology

The epidemiology of the hypopharyngeal and cervical esophageal cancer deals with the spread of the disease in the human population regarding sex, age, profession, time and space, as well as risk factors that contribute to these phenomena [5, 6].

The main factors involved in the occurrence of this type of cancer are chronic smoking and alcoholism. The risk of cancer occurrence is directly proportional to the ingested dose and alcohol concentration. The average age of onset is between 60 and 65 years, more common in men with a sex ratio of 5:1 men to women. The general tendency of the hypopharyngeal and cervical esophageal cancer is that of increased incidence, due to increased tobacco and alcohol consumption. Increased mortality is also associated with late diagnostic of hypopharyngeal and cervical esophageal cancer. 77.3% of patients are diagnosed with stage 3 or 4 upon admittance to the hospital [7, 8].

Usually, due to the anatomic relation between the site of the hypopharyngeal and cervical esophageal cancer, the two are studied together. Tumor lesions invade both regions at the time of diagnosis, which is usually in the late stages. At the beginning of the 21st century, hypopharyngeal and cervical esophageal cancer is still a major concern worldwide [8].

Piriform sinus location accounts for 85% of cases of hypopharyngeal cancer, 15% affect the posterior wall and the retro-cricoid region. The incidence of hypopharyngeal cancers varies from country to country and sometimes from region to region within the same country. The location of the tumor also differs from country to country and is closely related to the etiology factors involved. Hypopharyngeal and esophageal cancers are more common in countries with low social and economic standards and low education levels [3].

4. Pathology and pathogeny of hypopharyngeal cancer

The hypopharynx is lined entirely by a malpighian epithelium, so most cancers at this level are differentiated malpighian carcinomas (squamous cell carcinoma). However, hypopharyngeal cancer raises special problems for both pathologists and therapists due to its peculiarities, the way it spreads and the macro-microscopic aspects.

4.1 Morphopathology of hypopharyngeal cancer

From a macroscopic point of view, the hypopharynx may present two different forms of malignant tumors that are distinguished by their way of extension and prognosis. The ulcero-infiltrative form is most common and is characterized by invasion of the mucosa with more or less deep destruction of adjacent structures. The extension pathways mainly depend on the starting point of the tumor and the greater or lesser resistance of the encountered structures. The diffuse form with extension to the surface has a vegetative aspect being difficult to differentiate from an inflammatory type mucosa. This form develops on the surface without affecting the deep tissues being a carcinoma isolated to the mucosa but with distant spreading, affecting all or only parts of the epithelium of the hypopharynx. It is frequently associated with areas of infiltrative carcinoma and with more or less extensive areas of dysplasia and leucoplakia. There are other forms of cancer at this level with fairly well defined macroscopic and microscopic features: epithelial sarcoma (well-circumscribed tumor, pediculate, with minimal implantation surface, located especially in the membranous part of the piriform sinus and in the retro-cricoid region), wart-like carcinoma or malignant villous keratosis (rare, lymphophilic form, slow evolution, high chemo-sensitivity), adenoid malpighian carcinoma (muriform appearance, extremely rare, it can be found in the hypopharyngeal adenocarcinomas, non-Hodgkin's malignant lymphomas, melanomas).

4.2 Dissemination pathways

Tumor dissemination is achieved through direct local extension, lymphatic or hematogenous pathways. Finding the primary site and the pathway of dissemination is essential for the management of these tumors. Hypopharyngeal cancer is very rarely detected in the initial stage due to lack of symptoms.

Regarding local dissemination, tumors of the piriform sinus are located in its anterior angle from where the extension is made to the external and internal walls towards: 1. the internal wall of the sinus, from where it extends through the larynx (it is difficult to establish the pharyngeal or laryngeal origin of the tumor); 2. the lateral wall of the hypopharynx, from where it extends anteriorly to the anterior angle of the piriform sinus and the pharyngo-epiglottic fold, then to the thyroid cartilage and soft tissues of the anterior and superior cervical region to the lateral wall of the oropharynx.

The most important dissemination route is lymphatic. Lymph node invasion is present in 75% of patients at the time of diagnosis, detectable by palpation or imaging studies. For 10% of patients, lymph node involvement is bilateral from the time of presentation. Malignant tumors of the piriform sinus, lateral wall and posterior wall of hypopharynx usually spread towards the middle internal jugular lymph nodes. Tumors of the retro-cricoid region spread to the paraoesophageal, paratracheal and supraclavicular fossa [3].

4.3 Distant site metastasis

Distant site metastases are common. Patients with advanced cervical lesions and lymph node invasion are prone to develop distant site metastases to the lungs, liver, bones and brain.

5. Stages and grades

According to the American Joint Committee on Cancer (AJCC), the TNM staging of carcinomas originating in the hypopharynx is as follows (**Table 1**) [9].

6. Clinical and paraclinical evaluation of patients with hypopharyngeal cancer

Hypopharyngeal cancer is asymptomatic in the early stages, which is why most patients refer to a doctor in the advanced stages of the disease. The clinical examination corroborated with the paraclinical investigations contribute to positive and differential diagnosis. Histopathological examination is mandatory.

6.1 Symptoms

In early-stage tumors, symptoms are non-specific and may mimic laryngopharyngeal reflux or globus sensation. The first manifestation of the disease usually consists of unilateral dysphagia, especially during swallowing saliva. Very often patients go see a specialist due to the appearance of a cervical tumor or due to difficulty in breathing [10]. Dysphagia is progressive, initially for solid food and later for liquids. Severe dysphagia

AJCC Stage	Stage grouping	Stage description 2 cm = about 4/5 inches; 4 cm = 1.5 inches; 6 cm = about 2.3 inches
0	**Tis** **N0** **M0**	The tumor is located only in the top layer of cells lining the inside of the hypopharynx and has not grown any deeper (Tis). The cancer has not spread to nearby lymph nodes (N0) or to distant parts of the body (M0).
I	**T1** **N0** **M0**	The tumor has grown deeper, but it is only in one part of the hypopharynx, and it is no more than 2 centimeters (cm) across (T1). The cancer has not spread to nearby lymph nodes (N0) or to distant parts of the body (M0).
II	**T2** **N0** **M0**	The tumor has grown into more than one part of the hypopharynx, OR it has grown into a nearby area, OR it is larger than 2 cm but no larger than 4 cm across and has not affected the vocal cords (T2). The cancer has not spread to nearby lymph nodes (N0) or to distant parts of the body (M0).
III	**T3** **N0** **M0**	The tumor is larger than 4 cm across, OR the tumor is affecting the movement of the vocal cords, OR the tumor has grown into the esophagus (T3). The cancer has not spread to nearby lymph nodes (N0) or to distant parts of the body (M0).
	OR	
	T1 to T3 **N1** **M0**	The tumor can be any size and might or might not have grown into structures outside the hypopharynx, and it might or might not have affected a vocal cord (T1 to T3). The cancer has spread to a single lymph node on the same side of the neck as the tumor, which is no larger than 3 cm across (N1). The cancer has not spread to distant parts of the body (M0).
IVA	**T4a** **N0 or N1** **M0**	The tumor has grown into the thyroid or cricoid cartilage, the hyoid bone, the thyroid gland, or nearby areas of muscle or fat. This is also known as a **moderately advanced local disease** (T4a). The cancer has not spread to nearby lymph nodes (N0), or it has spread to a single lymph node on the same side of the neck as the tumor, which is no larger than 3 cm across (N1). The cancer has not spread to distant parts of the body (M0).
	OR	
	T1-T4a **N2** **M0**	The tumor can be any size and might or might not have grown into structures outside the hypopharynx (as far as a moderately advanced disease), and it might or might not have affected a vocal cord (T1 to T4a). The cancer is N2: It has spread to a single lymph node on the same side of the neck as the tumor, which is larger than 3 cm but no larger than 6 cm across, OR It has spread to more than one lymph node on the same side of the neck as the tumor, none of which is larger than 6 cm across, OR It has spread to at least one lymph node on the other side of the neck, none of which is larger than 6 cm across. The cancer has not spread to distant parts of the body (M0).

AJCC Stage	Stage grouping	Stage description 2 cm = about 4/5 inches; 4 cm = 1.5 inches; 6 cm = about 2.3 inches
IVB	T4b Any N M0	The tumor is growing into the area in front of the spine in the neck, surrounds a carotid artery, or is growing down into the space between the lungs. This is also known as a **very advanced local disease** (T4b). The cancer might or might not have spread to nearby lymph nodes (any N). It has not spread to distant parts of the body (M0).
	OR	
	Any T N3 M0	The tumor can be any size and might or might not have grown into structures outside the hypopharynx, and it might or might not have affected a vocal cord (any T). The cancer has spread to at least one lymph node that is larger than 6 cm across, OR it has spread to a lymph node and then grown outside of the lymph node (N3). It has not spread to distant parts of the body (M0).
IVC	Any T Any N M1	The tumor can be any size and might or might not have grown into structures outside the hypopharynx, and it might or might not have affected a vocal cord (any T). The cancer might or might not have spread to nearby lymph nodes (any N). The cancer has spread to distant parts of the body (M1).

Table 1.
Table 1.Hypopharyngeal cancer TNM staging according to the American Joint Committee on Cancer (AJCC).

and odynophagia are symptoms that occur in advanced cancers when the entire hypopharynx or cervical esophagus are invaded. Any unilateral dysphagia that persists for more than 2–3 weeks requires an ENT consultation. Weight loss is significant, sometimes leading to cachexia, so the assessment of nutritional status is an important element in establishing therapeutic management. Pharyngeal paresthesia, reflex otalgia, hemoptysis may be present. Dysphonia and dyspnea occur in late stages by the invasion of the pharyngo-laryngeal wall, recurrent paralysis or peritumoral inflammation [7].

6.2 Clinical examination

Inspection may suggest the condition by the presence of a cachectic patient, with the presence of a latero-cervical tumor or with anterior prominence of the larynx, hypersialorrhea and putrid breath. Performing bucco-pharyngoscopy we can detect synchronous buccopharyngeal cancers or tumor extension to this level.

The most reliable method of diagnosis in hypopharyngeal cancer is a direct examination of the pharynx and larynx so all structures can be assessed. Examination of the mucosa is mandatory and it can be done by using direct pharyngo-laryngocopy or fiber optic examination with or without digital image subtraction filters. Indirect pharyngo-laryngoscopy permits an overview of the tumor, its location and size, as well as the mobility of the vocal cords. Retro-cricoid tumors, as well as those located at the apex of the piriform sinus which is very difficult to highlight. Indirect signs like oedema, mucosal erythema, stagnant secretions or salivary stasis require further investigation (**Figures 1** and **2**).

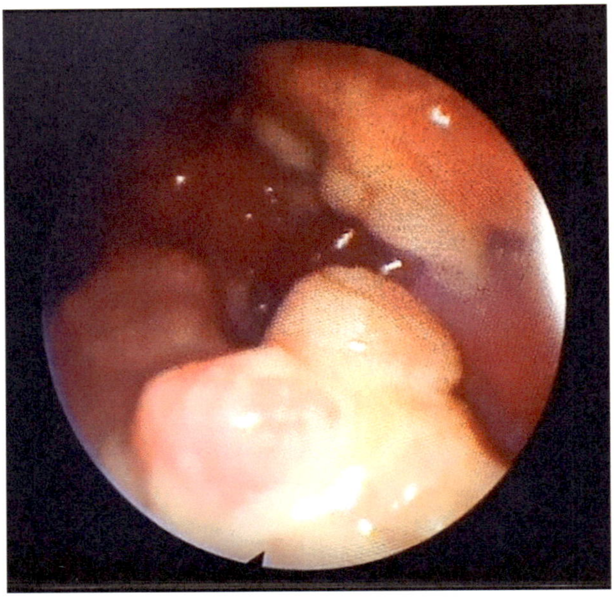

Figure 1.
Extensive tumor comprising all walls of the hypopharynx – circular tumor of the hypopharynx.

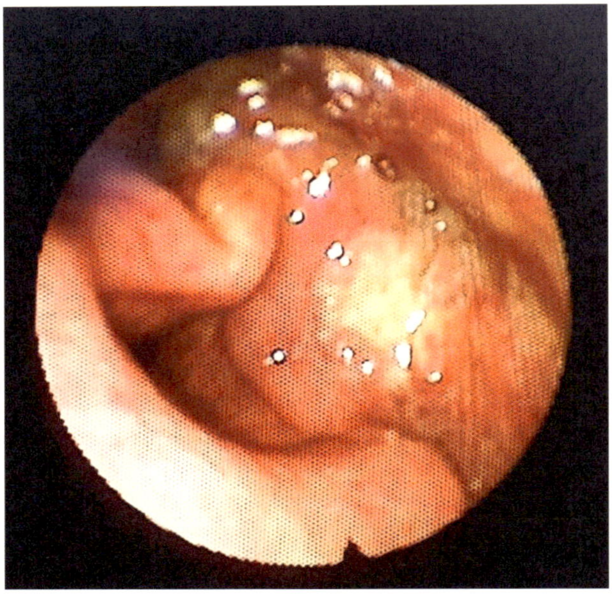

Figure 2.
Infiltrative tumor of the left pyriform sinus with the invasion of the left hemilarynx.

Palpation of the neck leads to the detection of metastatic lymph nodes. Spread towards cervical tissues through the mobility of the laryngeal skeleton can also be appreciated [11].

6.3 Paraclinical evaluation

To establish the correct and complete diagnosis, as well as to achieve the biological balance of the patient, the clinical examination must be completed with a paraclinical evaluation. Pharyngo-esophageal barium examination might reveal the location of the lower limit of the tumor and degree of extension. The main method of pre-therapeutic evaluation is computerized tomography scan (CT) with contrast which, compared to magnetic resonance imaging (MRI), provides us with important data related to cartilage invasion. Positron emission tomography scan and computed tomography (PET-CT) is to be considered mainly for stages III and IV, for the detection of the primary tumor, regional and distant recurrences, as well as for evaluation of oncology therapy response [3]. MRI helps to assess tumor extension to the submucosa, to the hyo-thyro-epiglottic fossa, paraglottic space, subglottic space and invasion of muscle tissue [12]. Rigid endoscopy performed under general anesthesia provides a clear view of the mucosa, determines the lower extension of the tumor and the relationship with the piriform sinus, upper esophageal sphincter and cervical esophagus and allows sampling biopsies in optimal conditions. Breathing and speech cannot be examined.

Since it is a cost-effective, non-invasive method of evaluating lymph nodes ultrasound examination is yet another imaging modality that has been recommended, but not preferred, for assessing the primary tumor site [13]. Chest CT scans or PET-CT are mandatory for the evaluation of distant site metastases. The therapy management plan is established by a multidisciplinary team. In addition, dental and nutritional evaluation should not be forgotten.

The only method that gives a certainty diagnosis is sampling biopsy during the endoscopic examination, followed by the histopathological examination and/or immunohistochemistry. Oncology therapy management, prognosis and follow-up must be determined by the tumor board [14].

7. Treatment of hypopharyngeal cancer

The treatment of hypopharyngeal cancer is complex, comprising a series of therapeutic methods consisting of surgery, radiotherapy and chemotherapy. These are applied successively or simultaneously, depending on the stage of the malignant neoplasm, but also on the general biology status of the patient [15]. For stage I and II cancers treatment consist of surgery or radiation therapy. Unfortunately, these patients are difficult to diagnose in stages T1N0 and T2N0 because of their lack of symptoms. Standard regimens of therapy for stages III and IV meaning resectable tumor include radical surgery followed by adjuvant radiotherapy and chemotherapy. Stage IV disease with the unresectable tumor benefits from elective treatment of radiotherapy combined with neoadjuvant chemotherapy [16, 17]. Unresectable tumors benefit from palliative surgical techniques (tracheotomy to maintain respiratory flow, gastrostomy for optimal nutrition). Neoadjuvant chemotherapy is used to reduce the volume of tumors and to convert them into operable or radiation-treatable tumors. It is used to treat patients with advanced local lesions to improve loco-regional control or survival [17, 18]. If the tumor has been converted by chemotherapy to a lower stage surgery will be performed according to the initial T! Psychological counseling of patients with hypopharyngeal cancer is mandatory both in the pre-therapeutic stage, during therapy and post-therapy.

7.1 Surgical therapy

The aim of the surgical treatment is to achieve a complete tumor resection with the preservation of functions as much as possible, minimizing a possible local or systemic recurrence. In some cases, the surgery is not performed either due to the invasion of the common carotid artery, prevertebral fascia or due to the lack of reconstruction possibilities or given by the functional status of the patient.

There are several types of surgery that can be performed:

- Suprahyoid pharyngotomy, indicated for tumors limited to the posterior wall of the hypopharynx. The reconstruction is done with a supported skin graft.

- Partial pharyngectomy, only for T1-T2 tumors limited to the posterior or lateral wall of the piriform sinus. It is not performed if the tumor is extended to the prevertebral fascia.

- Partial laryngo-pharyngectomy or extended supraglottic laryngectomy indicated in T1-T2 lesions of the piriform sinuses. It is not performed in patients over 60 years of age.

- Supraglottic hemi-pharyngo-laryngectomy, indicated in T2 cancer, is limited to the upper part of the piriform sinus. Both vocal cords are preserved, half of the ipsilateral wing of the thyroid cartilage is resected. Postoperative swallowing is possible. Removal of the tracheostomy tube is performed a few days after surgery. If chronic pulmonary aspiration occurs, a total laryngectomy will be performed.

- Posterior pharyngectomy is indicated in cancers located superiorly on the posterior wall of the pharynx.

- Endoscopic resection with CO2 laser does not require tracheotomy and reconstruction. It is performed in the case of T1-T2 tumors, but also the T3-T4 stages, but with a less satisfactory local control because of the narrow line of sight due to the use of a laryngoscope.

- Transoral robotic surgery (TORS) can overcome the limitations of CO2 laser surgery. It does not require tracheotomy and it is performed in T1-T2 stages, in some selected cases even T3. A Laryngeal Advanced Retractor System (LARS) to open the patients' mouths is required for achieving a proper exposure of the surgical site. Intraoperative extemporaneous histopathological examination is required to assess the invasion of the surgical margins [19].

- Total laryngectomy with partial pharyngectomy is indicated in T3/T4 tumors. It requires definitive tracheotomy and vocal rehabilitation.

- Subtotal laryngectomy, for tumors in stages T2 and T3 that pass through the apex of the piriform sinus and it fixates the ipsilateral hemilarynx. Patient will have permanent tracheostomy.

- Total eso-pharyngo-laryngectomy, indicated for tumors extending to the cervical esophagus. It is a combination of circular pharyngo-laryngectomy and total esophagectomy. Safety resection margins should be at 3 cm from the tumor edges.

- Total circular pharyngo-laryngectomy, indicated in cancer of the pharyngo-esophageal junction comprising the retro-cricoid region, the hypopharyngeal posterior wall and the cervical esophagus, T3-T4 stage tumors. Hypopharynx and larynx are completely resected circularly between the plane of the hyoid bone and that of the first tracheal ring, sometimes requiring inferior extension or extension to the thyroid gland [3, 4]. Reconstruction of the remaining defect is the difficult part of this intervention and requires the collaboration of the ENT specialist with the general surgeon and sometimes with the thoracic surgeon if the lower resection limit decreases in the upper mediastinum. Reconstruction is performed with musculo-cutaneous flap from the pectoralis major muscle, delto-pectoral tubular flap, free radial flap or jejunum-free flap, colonic transposition, revascularized fascio-cutaneous flaps, synthetic pharyngeal-esophageal prostheses.

As a first intraoperative stage after total circular pharyngo-laryngectomy a Montgomery tube can be placed between the pharyngostomy and the esophagostomy. In the ENT Clinic of Colțea Clinical Hospital in Bucharest, Romania, Professor Dr. Cristian Radu Popescu restored the pharyngo-esophageal continuity using a Montgomery esophageal prosthesis (**Figure 3**) [20].

This procedure has been used in patients without metastasis to the seventh lymph node station. The insertion of this synthetic prosthesis is done on the inside. The prosthesis is funnel-shaped at the upper pole and after adjusting the trusses of the esophageal and pharyngeal section to fit the ends of the prosthesis it is sutured at the base of the tongue and oro or hypopharynx with non-resorbable threads. The lower end of the prosthesis is inserted into the remaining esophagus over 5 cm. No suture is required at this level. The prelaryngeal muscles are fixed over the prosthesis. Postoperative feeding of the patient is performed by gastrostomy or by the nazo-gastric feeding tube inserted through the prosthesis at the moment of insertion. Because this method shortens and simplifies reconstructive intervention, without the esthetic defect left after flap reconstruction it has tolerance to radiotherapy comparable to other reconstructive methods, the material is biocompatible and allows the

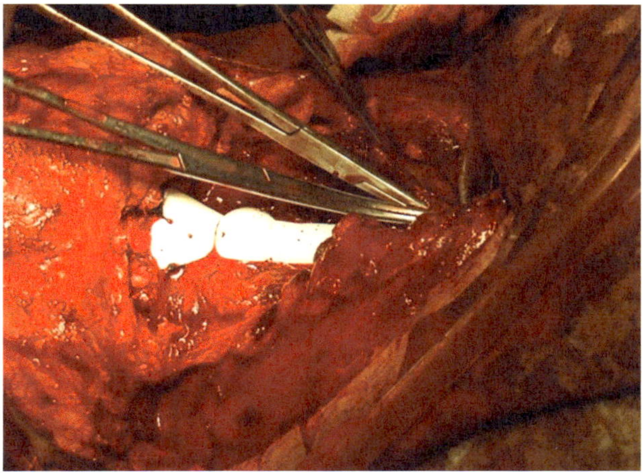

Figure 3.
Montgomery prosthesis is used for primary reconstruction of the upper digestive tract. The upper funnel-shaped portion of the prosthesis is sutured at the base of the tongue and the lower end is inserted in the esophagus.

resumption of oral nutrition. This method is now used as an alternative to reconstruction with flaps and not as a temporary solution [3].

Reconstruction of the defect can be performed with transposition of the small or large intestine in a mixed surgical team – ENT surgeon – general surgeon – vascular surgeon. This type of reconstruction favors a more natural feeding and deglutition process. However, it has more possible and life-threatening complications than primary reconstruction with Montgomery prosthesis (**Figures 4–7**).

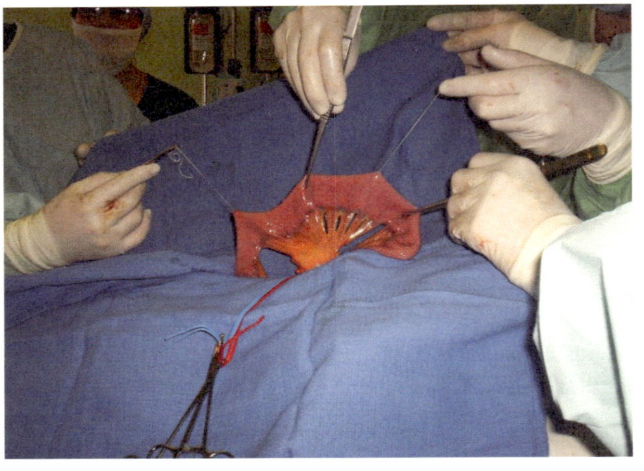

Figure 4.
Dissection and identification of a portion of the small intestine and vessel pedicle which will be resected and transposed to the neck area to reconstruct the upper digestive tract defect.

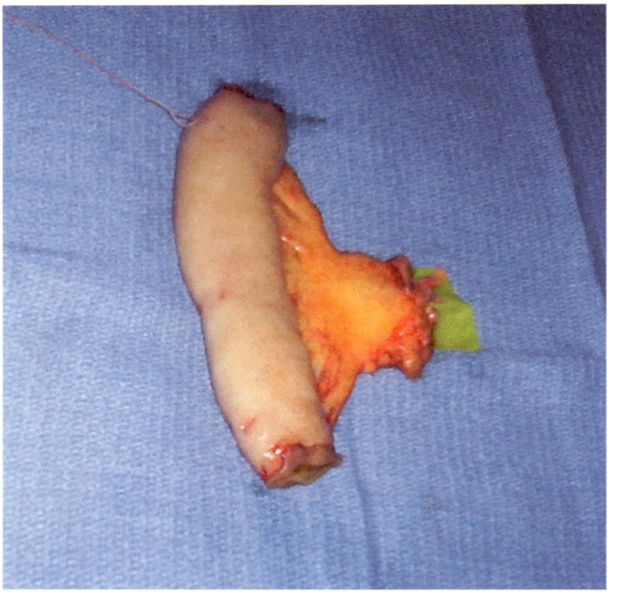

Figure 5.
Small intestine sample prepared for transposition.

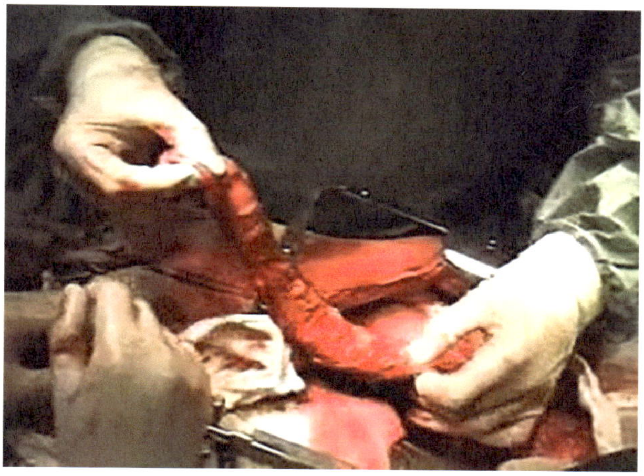

Figure 6.
Measuring the graft before suturing it in the neck region for reconstruction.

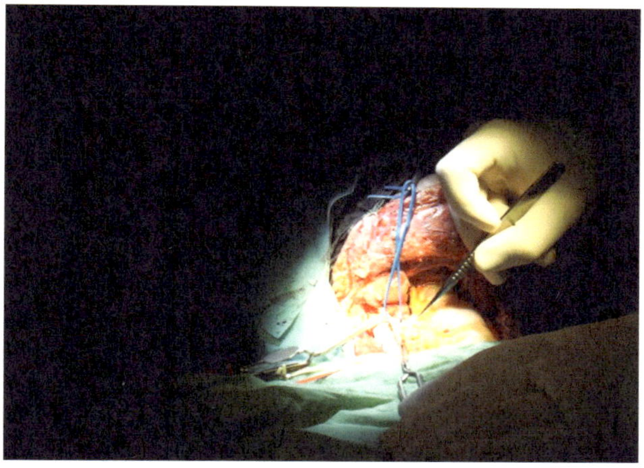

Figure 7.
Attaching vascular pedicle to the external carotid artery and internal jugular vein.

Oncological excision of the tumor must be accompanied by lymph node dissection, even if macroscopically metastatic lymph nodes. Micrometastases can occur in fatty tissue after complete resection. Neck dissection is done depending on the degree of lymph node invasion, but regardless of the N staging, station IV must be dissected if the pharyngo-esophageal junction is invaded [4].

There are four major types of neck dissection published by the Academy's Committee for Head and Neck Surgery and Oncology:

- Radical neck dissection – all lymphatic and fatty tissue are removed from the clavicle to the mandible, from the posterior edge of the trapezius muscle to the midline of the neck, spinal nerve, sternocleidomastoid muscle and internal jugular vein.

- Modified radical neck dissection – different from the previous one, either the spinal nerve (subtype I), the spinal nerve and internal jugular vein (Subtype II) are preserved, or the spinal nerve, VJI and SCM (subtype III) are preserved.

- Selective neck dissection – supraomohyoid, posterolateral, lateral and anterior.
- Radical neck dissection – in addition to radical neck dissection, other lymphatic structures are removed.

7.2 Radiotherapy

Radiotherapy as a single therapy is useful in T1 tumors, in rare T2 stage cases, in elderly patients, in patients who refuse surgery or as palliative treatment.

Radiotherapy in combined treatment regimens can be used before and after surgery. In our experience, the best treatment regimen is surgery followed by radiotherapy. Before radiotherapy, the patient needs a dental check-up to treat any conditions in this area, the treatment of comorbidities and the improvement of the general nutrition and biological status.

7.3 Chemotherapy

Chemotherapy is the treatment of hypopharyngeal cancer is used only in association with other methods of oncology therapy, not as a single way of treatment. Cytostatic drugs decrease tumor volume, improve clinical status and can prolong life. Adjuvant chemotherapy is instituted after surgical excision of the tumor and is used after or along with radiotherapy to eradicate a possible residual disease or micrometastases. Neoadjuvant chemotherapy is administered preoperatively to reduce tumor volume and primary tumor vascularization. It plays a role in lowering the chance of intraoperative tumor dissemination.

7.4 Nutrition

An important component in the therapeutic management of hypopharyngeal cancer is clinical nutrition. In hypopharyngeal cancer, we find a severe dysphagic syndrome that can lead to altered nutritional status, both by the cachexia-anorexia syndrome specific to the neoplastic disease, and by local causes that lead to weight loss and malnutrition. Tumor resection can cause severe disturbances to the complete cessation of food intake, and radiation therapy alters the taste and affects the surrounding normal tissues, compromising nutritional status.

Clinical nutrition can be achieved by the enteral or parenteral route. Enteral feeding is preferable in the case of a functional gastrointestinal tract and is made through the nasal-intestinal tubes (nasogastric, nasoduodenal or nasojejunal), stents mounted in the upper digestive tract, through the esophagostoma, gastrostoma or jejunostoma. The patient must learn to administer his own enteral nutrition, which can last for several months. If enteral feeding is not possible, the parenteral route of nutritional support is used, so that malnutrition does not compromise the surgery and the patient's life. Postoperatively, patients have a strict contraindication to oral feeding, and even swallowing saliva can adversely affect the prognosis by the appearance of fistulas. The nutritional intake is ensured on the nasogastric tube, gastrostoma, jejunostoma, nasojejunal tube. The nasogastric tube is kept for at least 10 days, depending on the reconstructive procedure used.

The nutrition of these patients includes a complete plan tailored to the condition of the patients and their nutritional status to reduce morbidity and mortality, being considered a method of adjuvant treatment with chemo- and radiotherapy in patients with hypopharyngeal cancer [3].

8. Prognosis

Hypopharyngeal cancer is asymptomatic in early-stage and patients go to a physician in advanced disease stages when metastases are already present and the prognosis is reserved. At the presentation, to the physician 50% of patients show cervical lymph node metastases. The survival rate in hypopharyngeal cancer depends on the tumor stage. Patients in T1-T2 stages have a survival rate at five years of approximately 60%. For patients in stages T3-T4 the survival rate decreases to 17–25%. Cancers in stages I and II, located on the posterior wall of the hypopharynx, have a much better prognosis compared to pyriform sinus cancers, even if it is small, but cause early metastases. Cancers of the retro-cricoid region are diagnosed in advanced stages with extended metastases at paratraheal and mediastinal sites with a severe prognosis. Patients with hypopharyngeal cervical esophagus cancer who have suffered reconstructions, have a two-year survival rate between 9 and 39%. The five-year survival rate in hypopharyngeal cancers is the lowest of cancers with other head and neck localizations [3].

9. Conclusions

Hypopharyngeal cancer mainly affects men around the age of 60. It is mostly located in the pyriform sinus, being a squamous cell carcinoma. Being asymptomatic in the early stages patients at the time of diagnosis are classified in stages III and IV of the disease, presenting cervical lymph node metastases and extensive tumors. Most patients require extensive surgical interventions and only a few can benefit from partial interventions. The type of neck dissection depends on the level of lymph node invasion. More than 50% of patients present local recurrences in the first five years after the surgical intervention, the risk of local recurrences being significantly higher in retro-cricoid and posterior wall tumors than in pyriform sinus tumors. The survival rate of hypopharyngeal cancer patients is influenced by tumor location and tumor stage. Therapy must be individualized, multimodal, with correct evaluation for each case and by involving several specialists like surgeons, radiotherapists, chemotherapists, nutritionists, psychologists. Surgical treatment remains the indication with the best results both as first intent and after radiotherapy failure, although it involves the sacrifice of the larynx. Montgomery pharyngoplasty after circular pharyngo-laryngectomy through the C. R. Popescu technique is a viable reconstructive alternative for oral feeding with small complications, low mortality rates and low hospitalization period. Surgery must be followed by radiotherapy and chemotherapy.

Conflict of interest

The authors declare no conflict of interest.

Author details

Oancea Alina Lavinia Antoaneta[1,2]*, Berteșteanu Șerban Vifor Gabriel[1,2], Grigore Raluca[1,2] and Popescu Bogdan[1,2]

1 General Medicine Faculty, ENT Head and Neck Surgery Department, University of Medicine and Pharmacy "Dr. Carol Davila" Bucharest, Bucharest, Romania

2 ENT Head and Neck Surgery Clinic, "Colțea" Clinical Hospital Bucharest, Bucharest, Romania

*Address all correspondence to: dr.alina.oancea@gmail.com

References

[1] Oancea ALA, Briceag I, Popescu CR. Extinderea indicațiilor chirurgiei cancerului laringian prin tehnici chirurgicale deschise – laringectomia orizontală supraglotică. Romanian Medical Journal. 2014;**61**(1): 64-67

[2] Scăunașu RV, Voiculescu S, Popescu B, Balalau C. The psychological influence of the diagnosis of breast cancer on therapeutic options selection. Journal of Mind and Medical Sciences. 2017;**4**(2):12. DOI: 10.22543/7674.42.P172177

[3] Berteșteanu ȘVG, Popescu RC. Cancerul de jonctiune faringoesofagiană. Reconstrucția protetică. 1st ed. Bucharest: Editura Universitară Carol Davila; 2012. DOI: 978-973-708-616-7

[4] Oancea ALA, Popescu CR, Bordei P. Cancerul de laringe. Corelații anatomo-chirurgicale. 1st ed. Bucharest: Editura Universitară Carol Davila; 2011. DOI: 978-973-708-597-9

[5] Popescu B, Bertesteanu ȘVG, Păun AO, Popescu CR, Balalau OD, Dumitrache P, et al. Differences Between Men and Women with Total Laryngectomy. Journal of Mind and Medical Sciences. 2015;**2**(2):100-107

[6] Popescu B, Popescu CR, Grigore R, Mogoantă CA, Ioniță E, Moculescu C, et al. Morphology and morphopathology of hypopharyngo-esophageal cancer. Romanian Journal of Morphology and Embryology. 2012;**53**(2):243-248

[7] Garneau JC, Bakst RL, Miles BA. Hypopharyngeal cancer: A state of the art review. Oral Oncology. 2018;**86**:244-250. DOI: 10.1016/j.oraloncology.2018.09.025

[8] Popescu CR, Bertesteanu ȘVG, Mirea D, Grigore R, Lonescu D, Popescu B. The epidemiology of hypopharynx and cervical esophagus cancer. Journal of Medicine and Life. 2010;**3**(4):394-401

[9] Amin MB, Edge SB, Greene FL, Byrd DR, Brookland RK, Washington MK, et al, editors. AJCC Cancer Staging Manual. 8th ed. New York: Springer International Publishing; 2017. DOI: 978-3-319-40617-6

[10] Hall SF, Groome PA, Irish J, O'Sullivan B. The natural history of patients with squamous cell carcinoma of the hypopharynx. The Laryngoscope. 2008;**118**(8):1362-1371. DOI: 10.1097/MLG.0b013e318173dc4a

[11] Hoffman HT, Karnell LH, Shah JP, Ariyan S, Brown GS, Fee WE, et al. Hypopharyngeal cancer patient care evaluation. The Laryngoscope. 1997;**107**(8):1005-1017. DOI: 10.1097/00005537-199708000-00001

[12] Jager EA, Ligtenberg H, Caldas-Magalhaes J, Schakel T, Philippens ME, Pameijer FA, et al. Validated guidelines for tumor delineation on magnetic resonance imaging for laryngeal and hypopharyngeal cancer. Acta Oncologica. 2016;**55**(11):1305-1312. DOI: 10.1080/0284186X.2016.1219048

[13] Fukuhara T, Matsuda E, Hattori Y, Donishi R, Ehara H, Fujiwara K, et al. Usefulness of ultrasound for assessing the primary tumor of hypopharyngeal carcinoma. Laryngoscope Investigative Otolaryngology. 2017;**2**(6):390-394. DOI: 10.1002/lio2.126

[14] Popescu B, Oașă ID, ȘVG B, Balalau C, Manole F, Domuta M, et al. Strategies to improve activity and results of the head and neck tumor board.

Journal of Clinical and Investigative Surgery. 2020;**5**(1):9-12. DOI: 10.25083/2559.5555/5.1/9.12

[15] Pingree TF, Davis RK, Reichman O, Derrick L. Treatment of hypopharyngeal carcinoma: a 10-year review of 1362 cases. The Laryngoscope. 1987;**97** (8 pt 1):901-914

[16] Gleich LL, Collins CM, Gartside PS, Gluckman JL, Barrett WL, Wilson KM, et al. Therapeutic decision making in stages III and IV head and neck squamous cell carcinoma. Archives of Otolaryngology - Head and Neck Surgery. 2003;**129**(1):26-35. DOI: 10.1001/archotol.129.1.26

[17] Lajtman Z, Manestar D. A comparison of surgery and radiotherapy in the management of advanced pyriform fossa carcinoma. Clinical Otolaryngololy and Allied Sciences. 2001;**26**(1):59-61. DOI: 10.1046/j.1365-2273.2001.00430.x

[18] Dubois JB, Guerrier B, Di Ruggiero JM, Pourquier H. Cancer of the piriform sinus: Treatment by radiation therapy alone and with surgery. Radiology. 1986;**160**(3):831-836. DOI: 10.1148/radiology.160.3.3737924

[19] Wang CC, Lin WJ, Liu YC, Chen CC, Wu SH, Liu SA, et al. Transoral robotic surgery for pharyngeal and laryngeal cancers – A prospective medium-term study. Journal of Clinical Medicine. 2021;**10**:967. DOI: 10.3390/jcm10050967

[20] Grigore R, Popescu B, Berteşteanu ŞVG, Nichita C, Oașă ID, Munteanu GS, et al. The role of biomaterials in upper digestive tract transoral reconstruction. Materials (Basel). 2021;**14**(6):1436. DOI: 10.3390/ma14061436

Chapter 6

Pharynx Reconstruction and Quality of Life

Paula Luiza Bejenaru, Raluca Grigore, Bogdan Popescu, Alexandru Nicolaescu, Mihnea Cojocărița-Condeescu, Catrinel Simion-Antonie, Gloria Berteșteanu, Anca Cirstea, Teodora Diaconu, Bianca Taher, Simona Rujan, Dan Popescu and Șerban V.G. Berteșteanu

Abstract

Patients who are diagnosed with squamous cell carcinoma of the pharynx have a first delayed presentation, with advanced stages of the disease. Therefore, they frequently require a multimodal approach—by surgery, radio, and chemotherapy. Due to anatomic spatial limits and particularities, therapy can imply large organ resection with difficulties in reconstruction. Nowadays, there is a paradigm shift in the management of this pathology, with significant first referral to oncology departments and initiation as the first line of treatment of radio/radio-chemotherapy. As a consequence, salvage surgery may be mandatory in some selected cases. The proposed chapter will address the oncological particularities of the pharynx, with a focus on the oro- and hypopharynx, ways of reconstruction after oncological ablative surgery of these segments, and impact on quality of life (QoL) index. Speech, respiratory, and deglutition rehabilitation of these patients is essential and will be a distinct topic. This paper will have the structure of a literature review with clinical examples of reconstruction from ENT and Head and Neck Surgery Department of Coltea Clinical Hospital, Bucharest. Reconstruction methods used in our clinic are regional flaps and biocompatible prostheses in advanced stages. QoL index in our clinic is assessed with questionnaires developed by the European Organization for Research and Treatment of Cancer – EORTC QLQ C30.

Keywords: pharynx carcinoma, oncology, deglutition, reconstruction methods, QoL

1. Introduction

The pharynx is the main structure, in addition to the oral cavity, shared by two organ systems. It is funnel-shaped, the upper end being wider and located just below the lower surface of the skull, and the lower end being narrower and located at the level of the sixth cervical vertebra. Its muscular-membranous integrity allows it to mediate several vital functions such as swallowing, air conduction, and voice production [1].

Performing surgical operations in the pharynx require delicate technique in order to preserve the physiology of the organ. Reconstruction of the pharynx is probably the most demanding task of the surgeon. Treatment for advanced *laryngeal and hypopharyngeal cancer* can cause anatomical and functional sequelae. Surgery aims at curing, but also keeping the organ's function. In tumors in which there is the need to remove the entire larynx or in cases of *hypopharyngeal tumors* with the need to remove the larynx, closing the remaining pharynx, in most of the cases done primarily, can be performed in two ways, cross-sectional or T closure. In *pyriform recess* tumors, a part of the pharyngeal wall is resected together with the primary tumor meaning that the pharyngeal remain is smaller, thus one should use the "T closure" technique or the flap [1, 2].

1.1 Oncological disease of the oropharynx - diagnosis

The pharynx, with its anatomical and physiological particularities, is an increasingly common site for head and neck malignancies, as apart from individual genetic characteristics, it is an often offended part of the human body—both infectious diseases and environmental exposure to risk factors (alcohol, tobacco intake) have a well-established cause—effect relation. On the other hand, as we have a better understanding of viral oncogenesis, human papillomavirus (HPV)—associated squamous cell carcinoma (SCC) of the oropharynx (OPSCC)—is nowadays a distinct entity from the traditional tobacco and smoking-related OPSCC [3].

SCC is the most common malignancy of the oropharynx, with a rate of 90% from all malignancies. It is an invasive epithelial neoplasm with degrees of squamous differentiation and with a high lymphophilia, as it may present with early and extensive lymph nodes metastases. Epithelial precursor lesions, especially erythroplakia, severe dysplasia, and carcinoma in situ (CIS) are involved in the development in patients with a history of tobacco and alcohol consumption. These tumors are aggressive, with a high disruption of cellular histology, invasion of lymphovascular space, neurotropism, and infiltration of other tissues such as muscle and cartilage. SCC can be keratinizing to nonkeratinizing and well-differentiated to poorly differentiated. HPV-associated OPSCC has a different histopathology with a lack of keratinization and mature squamous differentiation [3].

Other types of malignant carcinomas, with lower rates of appearance, of the oropharynx may include lymphoepithelial, salivary gland tumors, soft tissue tumors, hematolymphoid tumors, and mucosal malignant melanoma [3].

1.1.1 Clinical

Presentation is often in advanced stages, as the symptoms of early tumors are nonspecific. Mainly, dysphagia, foreign body sensation or pain in the throat, oral bleeding, referred otalgia, or neck mass may be patients' complaints. The presentation may also be as an unknown primary with an isolated nodal mass and no upper aerodigestive tract lesions or radiologic imaging [3].

After a thorough anamnesis, with emphasis on risk factors and social aspects, physical examination should have a great focus on the tongue (appearance and movement), tonsillar, fossae, retromolar trigone, soft palate (appearance and mobility), base of the tongue, vallecular, and pharyngeal walls. Inspection and especially palpation of the tongue base, tonsillar fossa, sensate testing, and an office endoscopy complete the examination. A complete head and neck investigation is mandatory for excluding synchronous cancers and bimanual palpation of the neck to assess lymph nodes [3].

1.1.2 Imaging

Precise evaluation and treatment plans require detailed imaging with a focus on soft tissues, vascular, and bony structures. Consequently, computed tomography (CT) and magnetic resonance imaging (MRI) are both used, either as one or complementary [3].

Positron emission tomography (PET) with CT can be useful for unknown primary, synchronous primary tumors and distant metastases. Limitations of these techniques are influenced by previous surgery or radiotherapy (RT), and it is not usually used for tumor staging [3].

Gray-scale and Doppler ultrasonography (USG) studies of the neck are useful tools for the evaluation of the lymph nodes. Fine-needle aspiration (FNA) can be done simultaneously for the purpose of establishing a histologic diagnosis [3].

Distant metastatic spread may appear in organs such as the lung, liver, skeletal system and brain, and CT of the lung and/or MRI of the abdomen are recommended [3].

1.1.3 Endoscopy

As an in-office procedure, oropharyngeal lesions biopsy can be performed if the site of the tumor is the tonsil or soft palate. FNA with USG of the lymph nodes may assist the diagnosis in selected facilities. On the other hand, when the site involves base of the tongue, inferior tonsillar, or posterior oropharyngeal wall endoscopy, with or without microscopic assistance may be the next step in the diagnosis. Pan endoscopy under general anesthesia is an important tumor evaluation and biopsy tool, and also can be used to rule out secondary malignancy [3].

1.1.4 Biopsy

Although frozen sections are close in accuracy to the final diagnosis up to 90%, the final treatment decision is based on standard histopathologic evaluation [3].

1.1.5 Testing for HPV or p16 and staging

Testing for HPV or its surrogate marker, p16 overexpression delineates tumor diagnosis and prognosis, and nowadays, the new system of staging developed by the American Joint Committee presents some differences between non-HPV-associated (p16 negative) and HPV-associated OSCC. The main ones are regional lymph nodes (N), with differences in pathologic N category, as metastasis in more than 4 lymph nodes stages in N2 disease [3].

1.2 Oncological disease of the hypopharynx - diagnosis

SCC of the hypopharynx and esophagus are head and neck rare afflictions (3–5% of head and neck HN SCC) with the worst prognosis, as they tend to present in late stages, with significant submucosal extension and a hard clinically and radiologically estimation of the disease. Organ-preserving protocols involve a slow rehabilitation, with high rates of complications, like stricture or impossibility of decannulation due to aspiration events. On the other hand, advanced tumors often require reconstructive surgery, with a multidisciplinary approach. Rarely, in 5% of the cases, other types of carcinoma, such as adenocarcinoma, sarcomata, and lymphoma can affect the hypopharynx [3].

In the etiology of the SCC of the pharynx, the most cited carcinogen is alcohol intake. Although HPV can be detected in hypopharyngeal cancers, there is no strong correlation between the diseases, until up to date [3].

Plummer-Vinson or Patterson-Brown-Kelly syndrome, which affects primarily women (85% of the cases) is a syndrome that is associated with postcricoid and upper esophageal carcinoma. It involves dysphagia, iron deficiency anemia, and the presence of hypopharyngeal and esophageal webs. Chronic irritation may result in hypopharyngeal webs with progression to carcinoma. Improved nutrition and prenatal care may decline the incidence [3].

1.2.1 Clinical

As it is stated before, patients with hypopharyngeal and esophagus usually present in advanced stages of the disease. Clinical examination may reveal dysphagia, neck mass, sore throat, hoarseness, referred otalgia, shortness of breath, hemoptysis, gastroesophageal reflux (GERD), or even asymptomatic. Also, these patients may present with weight loss and malnourishment [3].

The examination should focus on the mucosa of the aerodigestive tract for primary and synchronous cancers evaluation. Flexible endoscopy (**Figures 1** and **2**), as well as neck palpation, is mandatory [3].

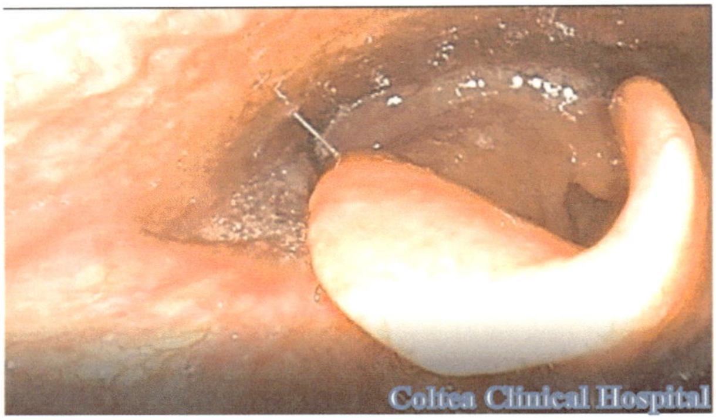

Figure 1.
Fiberoptic flexible view of the pharynx with hypopharyngeal carcinoma—note edema and saliva pooling.

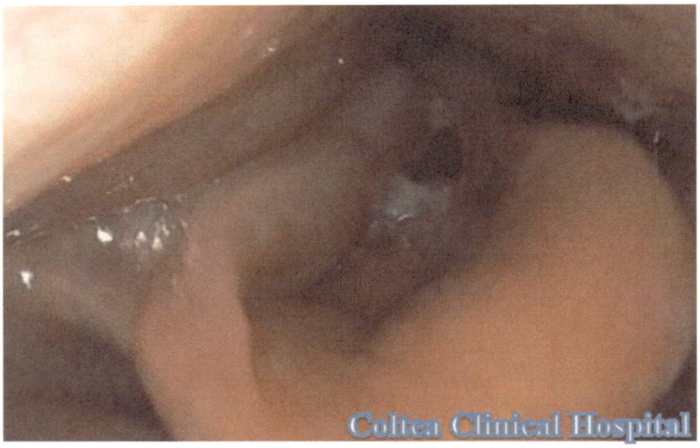

Figure 2.
Fiberoptic flexible view of the pharynx with hypopharyngeal carcinomas—note the laryngeal involvement.

Operative endoscopy, with complementary laryngoscopy and esophagoscopy are next steps in work-up. If it is possible, an assessment of second primary of the esophagus should be performed. Biopsy of the tumor is essential for diagnosis and further management. The pathology is usually SCC, but other rare lesions can occur: lymphomas, adenocarcinoma and neuroendocrine tumors, and thyroid malignancies with direct invasion; extremely rare: sarcomas, liposarcomas, angiosarcomas, and synovial sarcomas [3].

1.2.2 Imaging

Hypopharyngeal cancer has a particularity of submucosal spread that may be undetectable on clinical or radiographic examination. It is essential for the examination to focus on submucosal extension, involvement of the thyroid gland and metastasis to paratracheal and upper mediastinal lymph nodes, invasion of the prevertebral fascia, and carotid artery involvement as well. Cross-sectional CT or MRI is used for primary evaluation. CT is preferred as it assesses cartilage invasion. PET-CT is used for the detection of loco-regional recurrence and persistent disease [3].

1.2.3 Staging

Hypopharyngeal carcinoma and cervical esophagus carcinoma have different staging with appropriate treatment management (**Figure 3**). For hypopharyngeal tumors, involvement of the larynx, with fixation, is a sign of local significant spreading. For esophageal primary tumors, the assessment is based on the spreading of the layers of the esophageal wall [3].

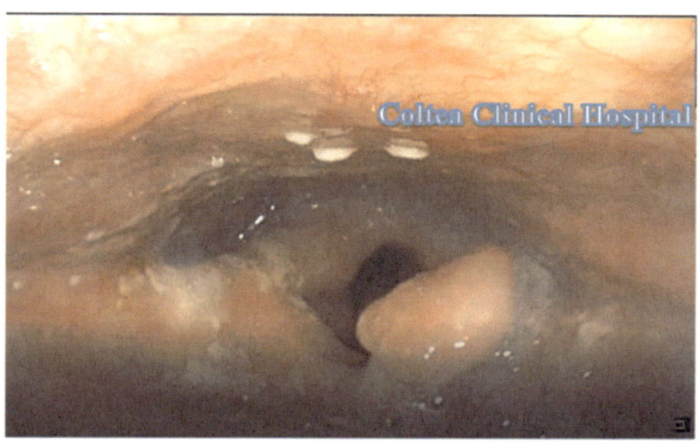

Figure 3.
Fiberoptic flexible view of the pharynx after base of the tongue carcinoma surgery and epiglottoplasty.

1.3 Treatment of pharyngeal carcinoma

Squamous cell carcinoma of the pharynx is defined by a late presentation, with the advanced stage that often implies submucosal spreading and early lymphatic metastasis. These characteristics predict a poor prognosis [4].

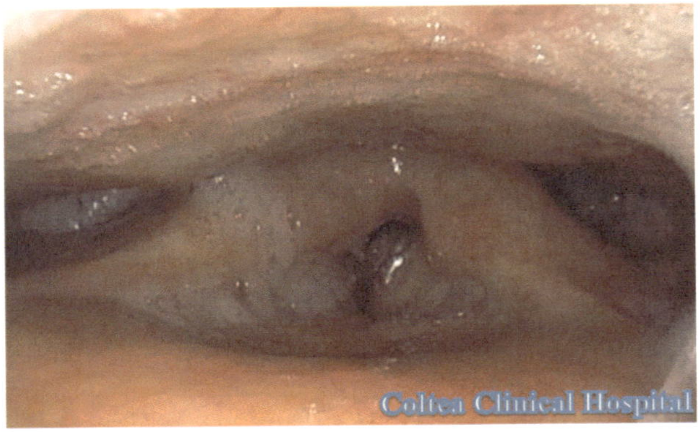

Figure 4.
Edema and mucositis after radiotherapy for oropharyngeal carcinoma.

In addition, along with scientific discoveries, new staging and ways of treatment appear and oropharyngeal carcinoma now requires tumor human papillomavirus (HPV) testing by p16 immunohistochemistry (IHC). Based on the result, there are clinical stages and consequently therapeutically differences. However, even in advanced stages, there is an indication of concurrent systemic therapy/RT (preferred in p15 HPV + T0–3, N3 or T4, N0–3), surgery (resection of primary with neck dissection), or induction chemotherapy followed by RT or clinical trials (**Figure 4**) [5].

Nowadays, stage-related ways of treatment begin to have a different angle, with organ preservation protocol with chemoradiation therapy and encouragement of conservation surgery that will maintain laryngeal functioning. Regardless, survival and oncological disease-free are mandatory and most patients diagnosed with hypopharyngeal carcinoma still need radical surgery—with total laryngectomy, partial of total pharyngectomy, and even esophagectomy. As a result, these kinds of surgeries are real challenges of reconstruction, especially when treating a circumferential defect [4].

Generally, it is well established that a residual mucosa bigger than 3 cm in width may grant a good primary closure. In other cases, a pedicled or free tissue transfer patch may be inserted. Reconstructive methods may include local flaps, myocutaneous flaps, free fasciocutaneous flaps, free jejunal interposition, gastric pull-up, and use of biocompatible materials—each with advantages and limitations. These are in straight relation with surgical team experience and resources [4].

There is a paradigm shift regarding pharynx carcinoma treatment and patients are discharged to trials of systemic therapy even in advanced stages. At present, advanced cancer requiring/amendable to pharyngectomy with total laryngecotmy (T1–3, N0–3; T1, N+) may have as a choice of treatment: induction chemotherapy, or partial/ total laryngopharyngectomy with neck dissection, thyroidectomy, and pretracheal and ipsilateral paratracheal lymph node dissection, or concurrent systemic therapy/RT, or clinical trials. After induction chemotherapy, complete response with stable or improved disease in the neck, NCCN guidelines recommend to go along with definitive RT or systemic therapy/RT. On the other hand, a partial response, depending on the nodal disease, means that the case may be treated with surgery or systemic therapy/RT. Advanced stages, with clinical T4a, N0–3 has as treatment of choice surgery, induction chemotherapy, concurrent systemic therapy, or admission to

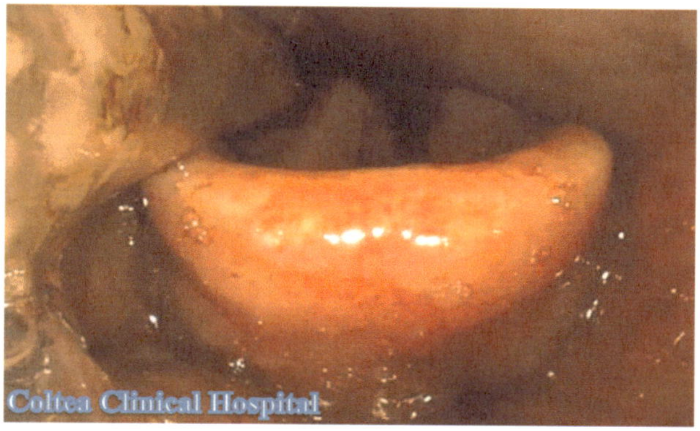

Figure 5.
Recurrent oropharyngeal carcinoma with bleeding—After surgical and RT therapy; note the presence of nasogastric feeding tube and the edema.

clinical trials. At follow-up, clinical changes will demand an adapted treatment [5] (**Figure 5**).

With treatment development, a variety of surgical skills and reconstruction techniques can deliver an adequate QoL for the patients, without certain differences between them. Even if different ways of treatment may seem even in oncological response, it is certain that salvage surgery is associated with additional complications (**Figures 6** and 7) [6]. Finally, patient selection and empowerment are critical in treatment and follow-up.

At the beginning, surgery of the upper aerodigestive tract malignancies presented a high rate of mortality (80%—Billroth's laryngectomies). As follows, surgical techniques advancement was necessary, taking into consideration that this kind of carcinoma affects two main vegetative functions, respiration and alimentation. Some authors elaborated an algorithm with treatment choices of defects of the laryngopharynx, hypopharynx, and cervical esophagus, with emphasis on complications of laryngopharyngectomy and back-up management [7].

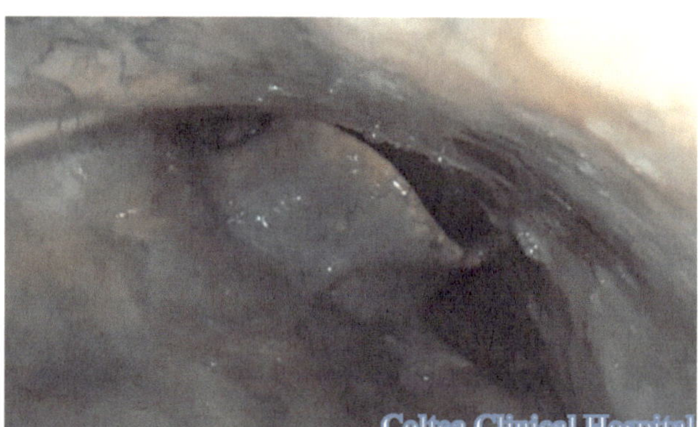

Figure 6.
Fiberoptic flexible view NBI assisted after hypopharyngeal carcinoma surgery with primary reconstruction.

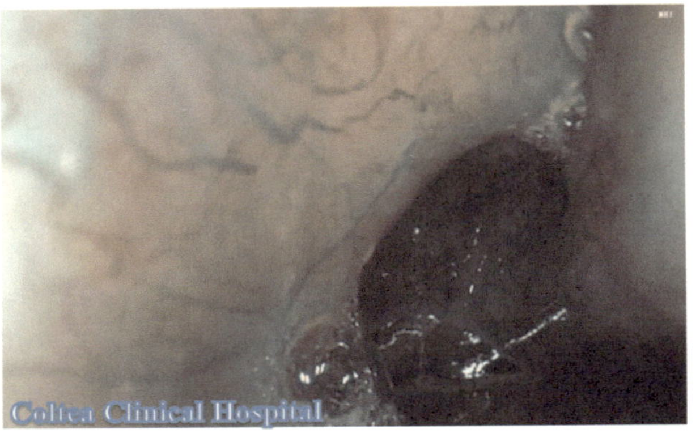

Figure 7.
Fiberoptic flexible view NBI assisted after hypopharyngeal carcinoma surgery with primary reconstruction. Close-up on the right reconstructed pharyngeal wall.

2. Reconstruction of the pharynx

Oropharyngeal reconstruction is a complex and difficult process that should perform a combined evaluation of the size, location of the defect, patient's age and comorbid status, and the use of the simplest reconstruction with the highest level of function. For small defects healing by secondary intention is the simplest way of approach; but with extensive lesions, the next steps in the reconstruction ladder should be primary closure, skin grafts, local and regional flaps, or free flaps (**Figure 8**) [3].

Hypopharyngeal defects often require a multidisciplinary approach and are associated with a high risk of mortality and morbidity—fistula development and vascular offense are the main concerns in this kind of surgery. Thus, the goals of reconstruction are the protection of the great vessels, restoration of the pharyngeal conduit, protection of the airway, and rehabilitation of the voice. Options for reconstruction are local and regional cervical skin flaps and deltopectoral, pectoralis, and latissimus flaps; gastric and colonic interpositions; and revascularized fascial and gastroomental autogenous transplants. Literature reviews conclude that vascularized tissue use has a reduced fistula rate, even when patient history includes RT. The decision must also be made in a ladder fashion and consider if the defect is partial or circumferential [3].

Certain milestones should be reached for an ideal hypopharyngeal reconstruction: single-stage procedure, high success rate for tissue transfer, low donor-site morbidity, low fistula and stenosis rates, restoration of the ability to speak and swallow, able to achieve a successful reconstruction in heavily radiated areas, and tolerance of postoperative radiotherapy [8].

In general practice, it is well established that a residual mucosa bigger than 3 cm in width grants primary closure. On contrary, a pedicled or free tissue transfer patch may be inserted [3].

In straight correlation with surgeon's experience, reconstructive methods may include local flaps, myocutaneous flaps, free fasciocutaneous flaps, free jejunal interposition, gastric pull-up, colon interposition, or even use of biocompatible materials—each with advantages and throwbacks, with a brief review in **Table 1**.

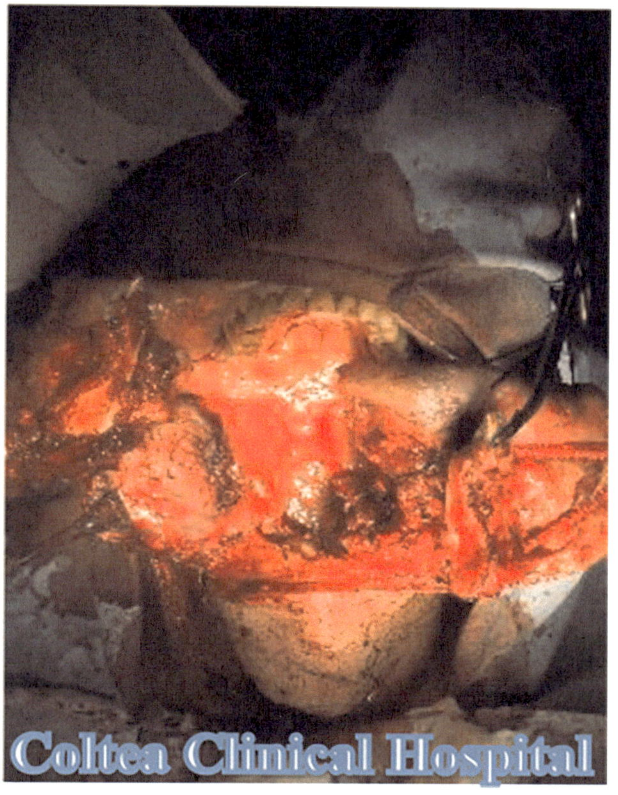

Figure 8.
Advanced oropharyngeal carcinoma—Trans mandibular approach.

Reconstruction	Advantages	Disadvantages
Primary closure, when possible	Decreased pain after surgery Less chance of secondary bleeding Superior speech and swallowing rehabilitation	Tension and contracture of the tissue Difficult surveillance over profound margins (than healing by secondary intention)
Local flaps	Optimal time management	Can be used for limited defects
Regional flaps	Single-stage reconstruction They can fill large defects—muscular bulks Do not require multidisciplinary teams Low donor site morbidity Fit for salvage surgery and patients with severe comorbidities—good time management	They can be too bulky, with high complication rates especially after oropharyngeal reconstruction They may require pedicle monitoring
Free muscular flaps	Low donor site morbidity Can be done in one stage surgery Tolerates well postoperative RT Superior speech rehabilitation	Multidisciplinary approach High complications rate: strictures or fistulas

Reconstruction	Advantages	Disadvantages
Free digestive flap interposition	Anatomical advantages Good vascularization Earlier deglutition rehabilitation	Dysphagia—uncoordinated peristalsis, dumping syndrome Difficulties in swallowing and voice rehabilitation Multidisciplinary approach Abdominal surgery complications
Biocompatible materials	One stage surgery and do not require multidisciplinary teams Optimal time management	Biofilms development High complication rates: fistula

Table 1.
Means of reconstruction after oncological surgery of the pharynx.

2.1 Local flaps

Healing by secondary intention can be used for defects less than 5 to 6 cm and it is not advisable when the pharynx communicates with the neck and after open procedures. When it is possible, this procedure is preferred from primary closure, as it can give oncological surveillance over profound margins and gives less tension and contracture. Primary closure has the benefits of decreased pain after surgery, less chance of secondary bleeding, and superior results in speech and swallowing rehabilitation [3].

For oropharyngeal reconstruction, local flaps may be used after open procedures. The palatal island, uvulopalatal, inferior and superior pharyngeal, the superior-constrictor advancement-rotation (SCARF), facial artery myomucosal (FAMM), and the buccinators myomucosal flaps can be considered as the main local flaps for oropharyngeal defects. These flaps can be used for limited defects [3].

2.2 Regional flaps

2.2.1 The pectoralis major flap reconstruction technique

The pectoralis major miocutaneous (PMMC) flap is an often used flap, with an excellent blood supply—from the pectoral branch of the thoracoacromial artery [4]. Its main advantages are single-stage reconstruction with muscle bulk, which is important in filling large defects; it can be rapidly raised from the anterior chest wall and it does not require multidisciplinary teams, with additional expertise in microvascular or abdominal surgery, the morbidity of the donor site is low, and with high importance, it comes from a nonirradiated area in salvage surgery. However, this flap seems to be too bulky, and after reconstruction some authors report high fistula and stricture rates. Still, it is a helpful choice for salvage surgery, for elderly patients and for patients with severe comorbidities—when time management needs to be optimal [4].

The pectoralis major muscle is a thick, fan-shaped muscle, that lies underneath the breast tissue. It has three parts of origin, a clavicular one, at the anterior surface of the medial half of the clavicle, a sternocostal one on the anterior surface of the sternum and the first seventh costal cartilages, and one abdominal at the level of the right abdominal muscle sheath. The insertion is made through a common tendon formed by the three parts of origin at the intertubercular sulcus of the humerus [9].

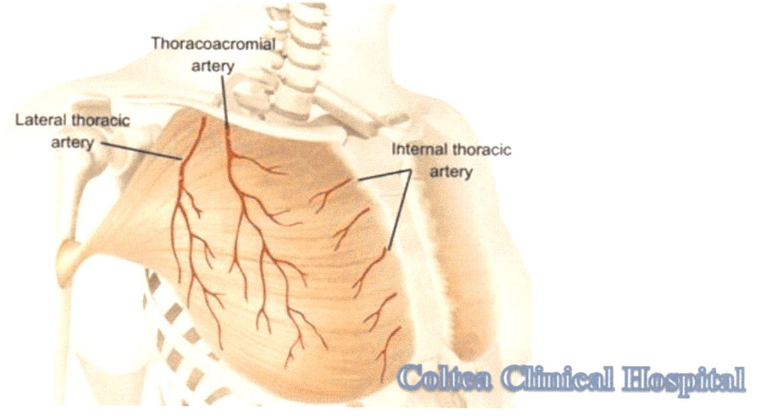

Figure 9.
Arterial supply of the pectoralis major muscle.

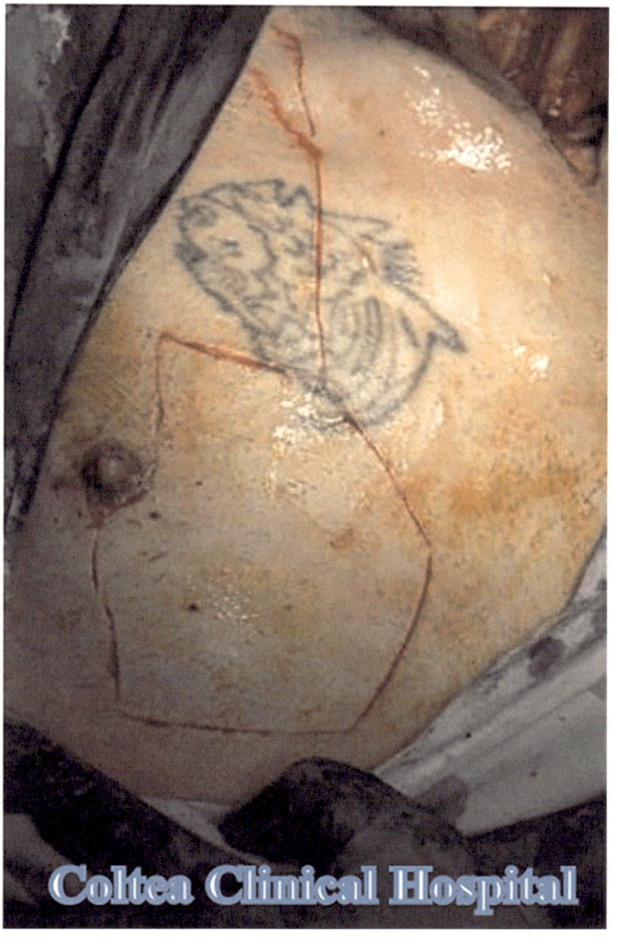

Figure 10.
Skin island and vascular pedicle of the PMMC.

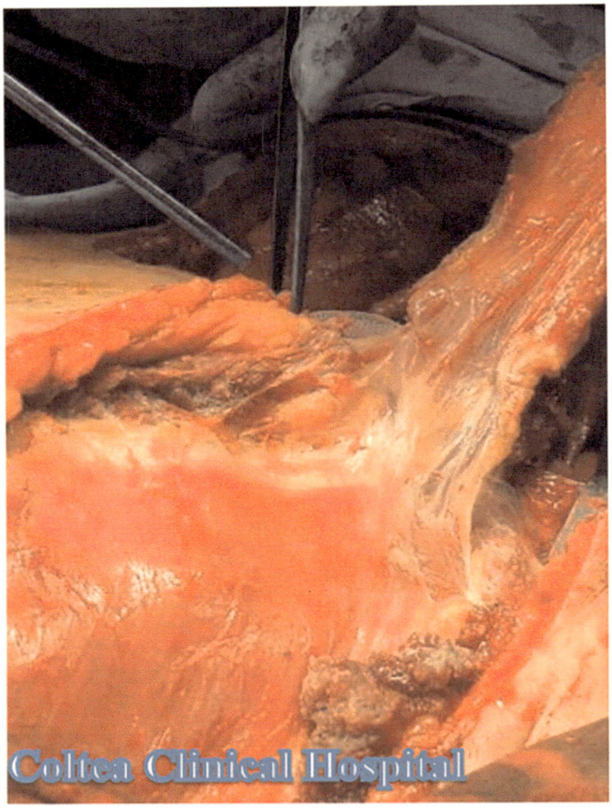

Figure 11.
Skin island and vascular pedicle of the PMMC.

It is a superficial muscle, being covered by skin, subcutaneous connective tissue, the medial and intermediate supraclavicular nerves, and the mammary gland. It covers the small pectoralis, anterior serratus, subclavius muscles, ribs, and intercostal spaces. The close relationship with the pleura must be taken into account when harvesting the flap.

The arterial supply of the pectoralis major is provided by the pectoral branches of the thoracoacromial artery, the perforating branches of the internal thoracic artery, and the perforating branches of the lateral thoracic artery (**Figure 9**). Its venous drainage is through the pectoral vein, which drains into the subclavian vein [10, 11].

The first step when using a chest flap for reconstruction is to determine the length of the flap required. A dry gauze is used to perform the measurement. This is placed on the middle of the collarbone, this being the place where the pectoral flap will be rotated. The upper limit of the flap is measured, and then the gauze is pivoted lower to establish the lower edge of the flap. The boundaries of the skin tissue island are achieved by drawing a line from the acromion to the xiphoid process. A second line is drawn perpendicular to the clavicle at the intersection of the lateral third with 2/3 medial of the clavicle. The intersection of the two lines represents the upper limit of the skin islet. The lower limit of the skin island is represented by the 7th rib, the lateral one is the extremity of the pectoralis major muscle, and the medial one is the middle sternum (**Figure 10**). Preferably, the island should have an elliptical shape to facilitate closure [12].

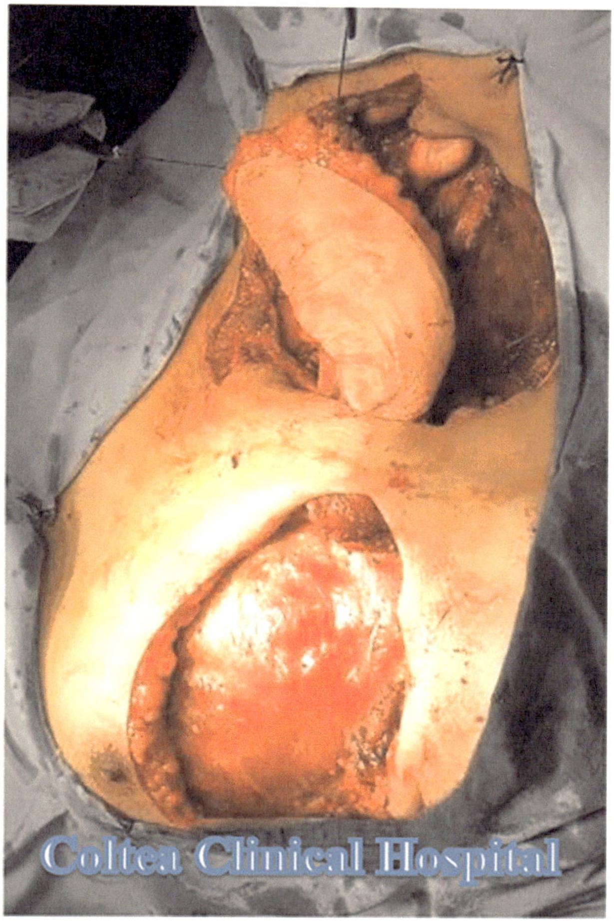

Figure 12.
Transposition of the flap and compression dressing with 2 catgut.

The next step is to expose the large pectoralis muscle. The dissection is performed from medial to lateral. After exposing the pectoralis major muscle, its edge is sutured to the subcutaneous connective tissue of the skin island. An incision is then made from the medioclavicular level to the myocutaneous island. Lifting of the flap is done by digital dissection, deep to the pectoralis major muscle.

Dissection of the vascular pedicle must be done carefully so as not to damage it and compromise the flap. It is recommended to leave an equal thickness of tissue around the flap (**Figure 11**).

A subcutaneous tunnel is made at the level of the clavicle through which the flap is transposed at the level of the defect (**Figure 12**). A drain is placed at the level of the pectoral defect, at a distance from the vascular pedicle. The suture is made in 2 planes. A compression dressing is held in place for 2 days (**Figure 13**).

Most often, reconstruction of the hypopharynx with the PMMC is performed after total laryngectomy. Because the posterior wall of the larynx is attached to the anterior wall of the pharynx, a significant part of the pharyngeal wall may be excised during total laryngectomy. If it is necessary to reconstruct the entire circumference of the pharynx, it is recommended to use a free flap (tubularized anterolateral tight, radial

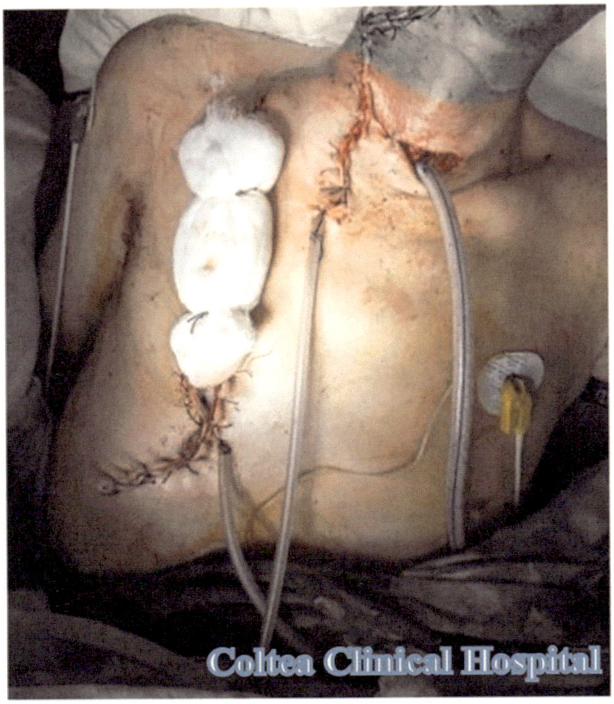

Figure 13.
Transposition of the flap and compression dressing with 2 catgut.

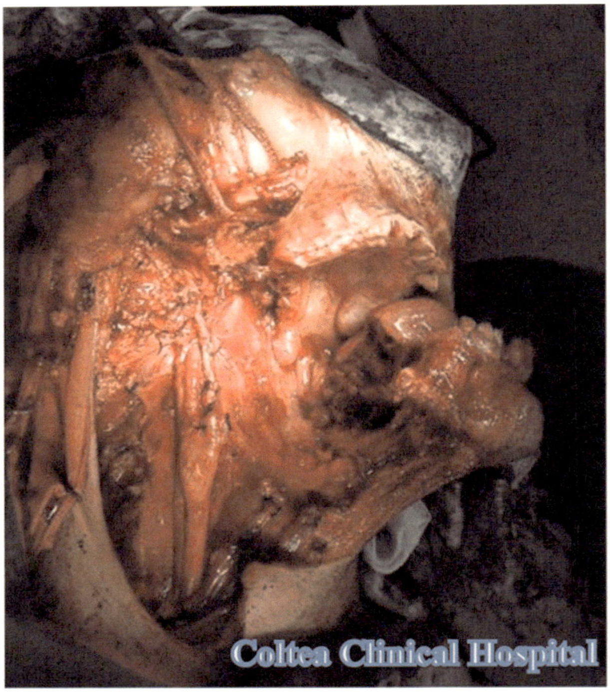

Figure 14.
Gigant oropharyngeal and cervical defect which needed PMMC reconstruction.

forearm fasciocutaneous free flap or jejunum). Defects of the pharynx extending below the clavicle are most commonly reconstructed with a gastric pull-up or colon interposition flap.

After harvesting and lifting the flap at the neck level using the technique described above, the flap is rotated 180 degrees to bring the skin side in. The closure of the defect begins at the caudal extremity of the pharynx. The right edge of the remaining pharynx is sutured to the left edge of the flap with 2–0 catgut sutures. Reconstruction of the pharyngoesophageal defect is done in the form of a racquet. A nasogastric feeding tube is inserted and passed into the distal esophagus before complete closure of the pharyngeal defect [13].

When an anterior cervical soft tissue defect is also present, a prelaminated pectoralis major pedicled flap can be used for reconstruction. This flap can provide two epithelial surfaces. This is a two-step procedure that involves first implanting a skin graft under the pectoralis major muscle. After maturation of the added tissue, the myocutaneous flap is transferred onto the neck, where the grafted surface is used for pharyngeal lining [14].

PMMC is also used for the reconstruction of defects of the oropharynx (**Figures 14** and **15**), but with a rather high complication rate. Complications include partial necrosis and less often total necrosis and fistula development. Due to the gravitational force, as it is a heavy flap, has a tendency to pull away, causing separation of the suture line, especially at the superior edge.

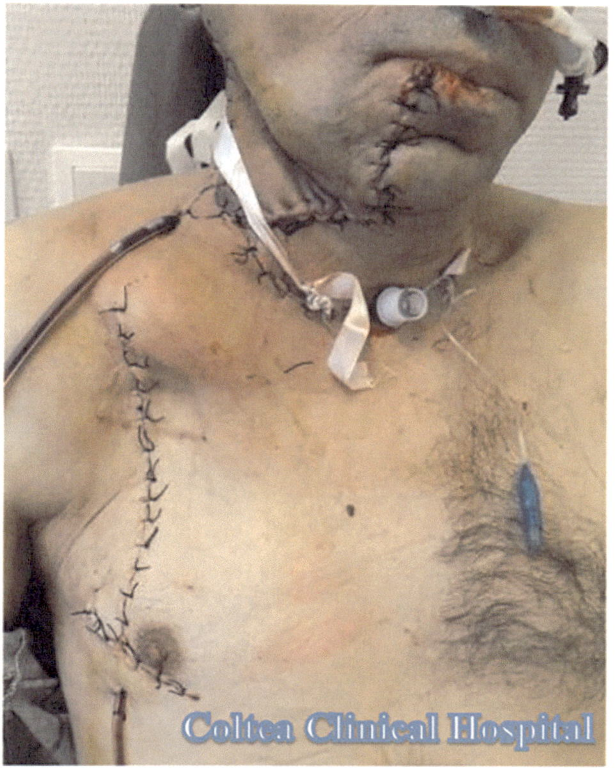

Figure 15.
Appearance of the patient 2 days after PMMC reconstruction for extensive pharyngeal resection and cervical region defect.

2.2.2 The sternocleidomastoid (SCM) flap

The sternocleidomastoid (SCM) is used as a pedicled flap in head and neck reconstruction since 1908, and although it has been previously associated with high complication rates, recent reviews state that preservation of the vascular pedicles and techniques improvements make it an adequate choice, especially when free flap surgery is inappropriate [15].

The muscle originates from the upper edge of the sternal manubrium, from the medial quarter of the upper face of the clavicle; the two muscle heads merge into a single muscle belly that is directed upwards and laterally. Insertions arrive at the mastoid process of the temporal bone and at the anterior portion of the superior nuchal line. SCM has fibers arranged in parallel; it is not a pennate muscle. The sternomastoid portion is the muscle area that develops a greater percentage of contractile strength than the other portions [16].

The arterial supply is given by branches of the external carotid artery (occipital artery and superior thyroid artery), which can be palpated, feeling the heartbeat in the medial-anterior portion of the muscle. The external jugular vein passes inferiorly and posteriorly the SCM, from which it drains venous blood (external posterior jugular vein and anterior jugular vein) [16]. Superior and middle pedicles are the most important to be preserved, as they give the major blood supply to the muscle. The inferior pedicle is the most controversial, with variations of origin—suprascapular artery, thyroid artery, or transverse cervical artery, and it cannot be relied on to perfuse the entire muscle. Some studies conclude that preserving the superior thyroid arteriovenous system is critical for the survival of the flap. Also, care to be taken to external jugular vein, as venous limitations may also affect flap viability [15].

Anatomic studies suggest that only one pedicle may not be not enough, as ischemic complications may appear due to a low vascularization in the distal end of

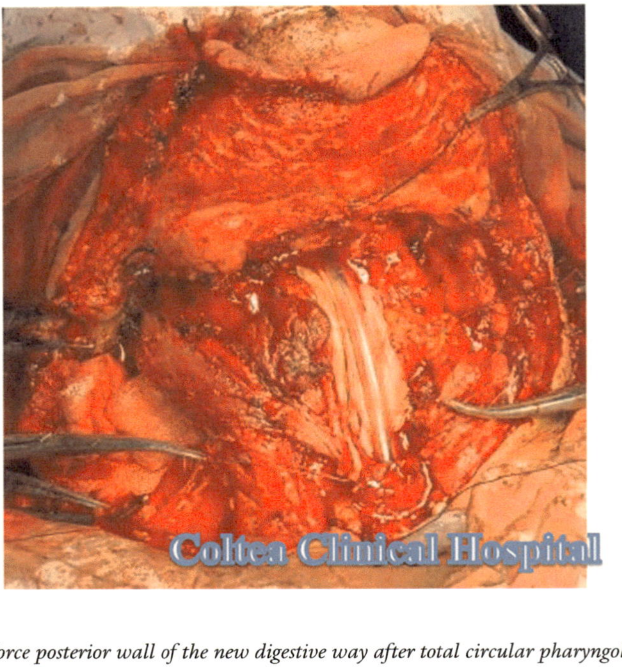

Figure 16.
SCM flap used to enforce posterior wall of the new digestive way after total circular pharyngolaryngectomy.

the muscle and some authors advocate the use of superior and middle pedicle, with dissection at the highest length to allow flap rotation. Single-headed SCM flaps can repair soft tissue defects up to 8 cm × 6 cm, and if a bone is needed an SCM flap with a clavicular bone graft can fix mandibular defects up to 6 cm long. The skin incision should be parallel to the muscle from the angle of the mandible, and with a clear view of the occipital and superior thyroid arteries. Skin platysma flaps are raised anterior to posterior to the SCM and muscle should be raid with its investing fascia. Separation from its superior or inferior bony attachments is done with a combination of blunt and sharp dissection. After flap harvesting, selective functional neck dissection can be performed. Suturing the skin on the muscle may be favorable for skin perfusion as it decreases tension and avoids tearing of the delicate perforators to the skin [17].

With a high versatility in head and neck reconstruction, this regional pedicled flap can be used as a myocutaneous, myofascial, myoperiosteal, or osteaomuscular flap. This flap is best used for defects below the level of the zygomatic arch. It is not advisable to use this flap if the tumor directly invades the muscle or if the neck dissection cannot be done adequately in order to preserve the pedicles, as oncological safety is the priority. The history of radiation is not an absolute contraindication [18] (**Figure 16**).

2.2.3 The supraclavicular (SC) flap

The supraclavicular flap is a versatile fasciocutaneous flap designed along the axis from the supraclavicular fossa extending over the shoulder. It is useful in the reconstruction of a variety of head and neck defects and can be ideal for pharyngeal and esophageal reconstruction [19].

Key anatomic landmarks are the SC triangle with identification of the cutaneous perforator of the supraclavicular artery. The supraclavicular flap is an elongated ellipse over the supraclavicular region with an inferior extension to the deltoid tip. It

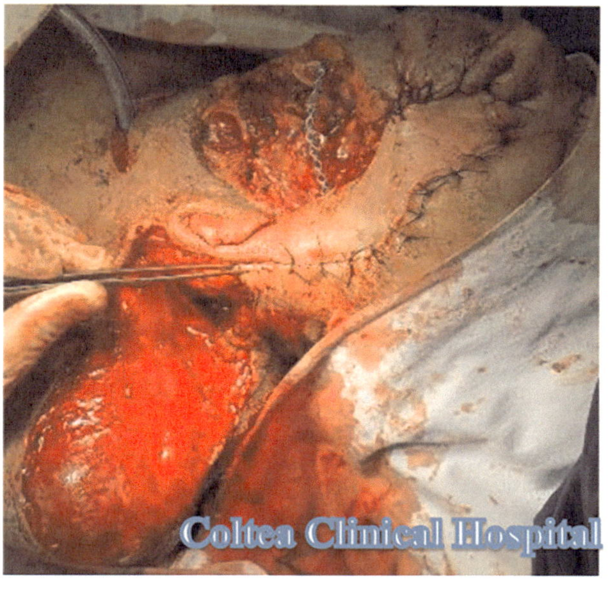

Figure 17.
Supraclavicular flap for oral cavity reconstruction.

can cover up to 8 cm of the defect. Flap elevation is done from distal to proximal, in a subfascial plane, and care should be taken to avoid injury of the cephalic vein on the ventral surface. Donor site can be closed primarily and drain placement is recommended (**Figure 17**) [18].

2.3 Multidisciplinary approach: Free flaps and other types of reconstruction

This kind of approach requires a multidisciplinary team, and the head and neck team must determine the approximate size of each tissue needed for reconstruction, thus communication is vital. Time management, especially when using tourniquets and gentle dissection of an intact vascular pedicle, is also of great importance. In addition, topical measures can assure viability: copious micro-irrigation with saline or heparinized lidocaine (2% lidocaine, 100 U/ml heparin) and papaverine irrigation (30 mg/mL). The free flap paddle should be manipulated while having a native supply. A delicate microsurgical technique and good pedicle geometry are the most important factors in microvascular anastomosis. The end-to-end anastomotic technique is the most commonly used. Postoperative monitoring is essential and visible flap inspection with pinprick can be supplemented by digital palpation and Doppler monitoring [3].

2.3.1 Radial forearm free flap

Radial forearm-free flap is considered the best choice for near-total laryngopharyngectomy defects, with high advantages, especially in tailoring options. Likewise, it has low donor site morbidity and can be harvested in one-stage surgery. It tolerates well postoperative radio-therapy and has seemed to have superior speech rehabilitation. As disadvantages, some authors report high complications rate, with stricture or fistula but which are manageable with conservative measures [20].

2.3.2 The free jejunal flap

In esophageal involvement, the free jejunal flap is a reliable way of reconstruction, with certain anatomical advantages. It is stated that up to 20 cm of jejunum can be harvested and as it comes along with the vascular mesentery, that allows obliteration of possible defects and protect the vascular structures of the neck. Deglutition rehabilitation seems to be earlier, but it may present with dysphagia because of uncoordinated peristalsis. Flaws of this flap are the quality of voice rehabilitation with excessive mucus production, the need for a microvascular reconstructive team, and in addition, abdominal surgical complications [21].

2.3.3 Gastric pull-up reconstruction

Gastric pull-up reconstruction is a surgical technique in which the stomach is brought, through the mediastinum to the neck along with the entire esophagus. The main indication for this procedure is esophageal carcinoma, with thoracic segment involvement. The main advantages are a great vascularization, with pedicle on the right gastric and gastroepiploic vessels, only one anastomosis is needed, one-step procedure, and the lowest stricture rate of all flaps. On the other hand, it presents high morbidity and mortality, with an overall incidence of complications of between 26% and 55%. Mediastinitis, difficulties in swallowing and voice rehabilitation, dumping syndrome are the main concerns postoperatively [4].

2.4 Transoral surgery techniques

As transoral surgery evolved, with even robotic-assisted (TORS), reconstructive ways for oropharyngeal defects should take into consideration structural features, such as creating an anatomic barrier between the neck and the pharynx and to ensure adequate coverage of the carotid artery. Functional considerations are restoring swallowing function, preserving speech and articulation, preventing aspiration, and maintaining velopharyngeal competence. Some authors created an algorithm that submits the factors determining more advanced reconstructions: number of subsides involved, exposure of the great vessels, communication with the neck, size of the defect (palate, tongue base), and radiation history. In defects with >50% of palatal defect, pharyngocervical communication and exposed carotid artery, after transoral robotic surgery, the authors recommend considering regional or free flaps [22].

Other authors found ingenious ways in TORS reconstruction, direct transposition of the ipsilateral naso-septal flap into the oropharynx via a trans palatal tunnel at the hard-soft palate junction [23].

As most centers and surgeons use more than one technique in reconstruction for hypopharyngeal carcinoma, multiple factors play in flap choice. Risk and benefit analysis is extremely important, especially for patients with circumferential loss of the pharyngoesophagus. Skin flaps have less donor morbidity than visceral flaps but are limited in obese patients. Free flaps need longer operative time but provide larger and more adaptable paddles for reconstruction [19] (**Figure 18**).

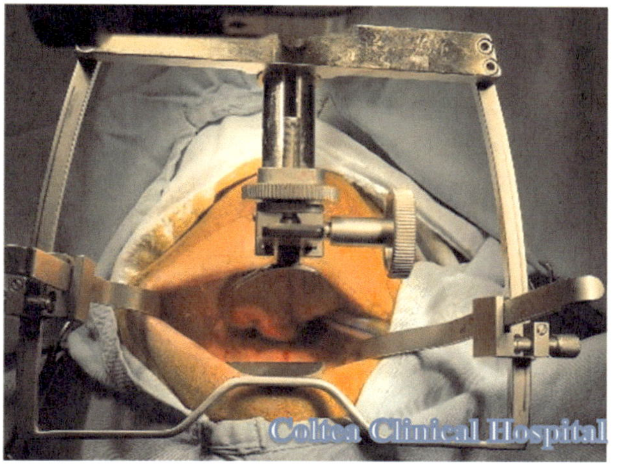

Figure 18.
Transoral surgery setup for base of the tongue carcinoma.

2.5 Biocompatible materials

A possible alternative in reconstruction for esophageal defects can be Montgomery salivary bypass tube. Precisely, this tube has two spherical zones which enable better stability and optimal saliva leaking along of tube, regardless of the head and neck position. Silicon rubbers used in prosthesis construction are the most appropriate solution in terms of morbidity, biocompatibility, functionality, and bacterial and fungal biofilm formation. A study conducted in "Coltea" Clinical Hospital, ENT department, Bucharest, concluded that insertion of a bacteriostatic agent, such as silver nanoparticles, decreases the fatigue strength, increases flexibility, and offers an optimal local protection solution against fungi development [6] (**Figures 19** and **20**).

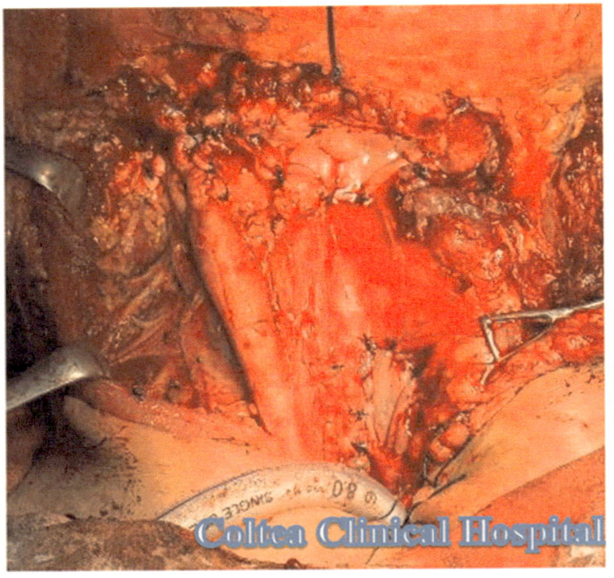

Figure 19.
Total circular pharyngolaryngectomy with radical neck dissection (note the carotid artery) and reconstruction with Montgomery salivary tube.

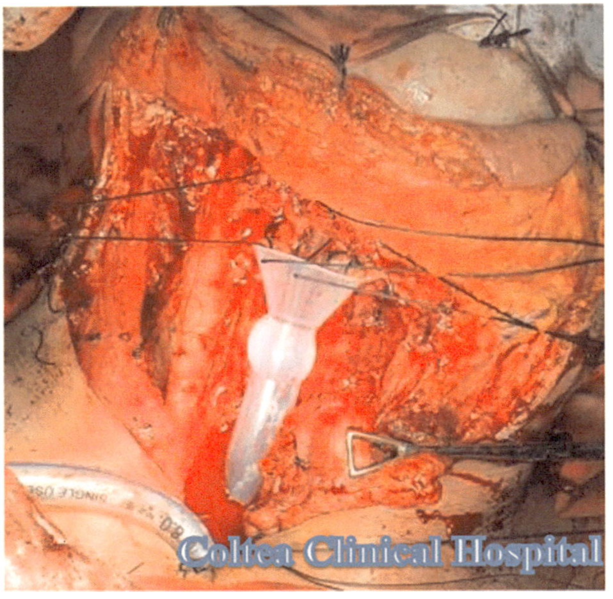

Figure 20.
Total circular pharyngolaryngectomy with radical neck dissection (note the carotid artery) and reconstruction with Montgomery salivary tube.

3. Improving QoL and rehabilitation

3.1 QoL after reconstructive surgery

The European Organization of Research and Treatment of Cancer (EORTC) QoL questionnaire (QLQ) is an integrated system for assessing the health-related QoL (HRQoL) of cancer patients participating in international clinical trials. The core questionnaire, QLQ-C30, is composed of both multi-item scales and single-item measures. These include five functional scales, three symptom scales, a global health status/QoL scale, and six single items. Each of the multi-item scales includes a different set of items—no item occurs in more than one scale. All of the scales and single-item measures range in score from 0 to 100. A high scale score represents a higher response level. The scaling technique described above is based upon the widely applied Likert method of summated scales, in which the constituent items within each scale are simply summed. This makes several assumptions about the nature of the items, the most important of which are (a) that it is appropriate to give equal weight to each item, and (b) that each item is graded on a linear or equal-interval scale. The raw QLQ-C30 scores can be transformed into scores ranging from 0 to 100 [24].

Swallowing, mastication, and speaking are major factors that affect the HRQoL of patients one year after operation for pharyngeal cancer. Some authors advocate that flap reconstruction after oropharyngeal cancer surgery can improve patients' QoL postoperatively [25]. Furthermore, there are studies that conclude that still surgery should be considered as a first-line therapy for oropharyngeal cancer because the surgery-based group achieved equivalent treatment outcomes and slightly better QOL scores than the RT-based group [26].

If the cancer is diagnosed in the late stages, disfigurement, chewing, speech, and shoulder function can be significantly below the preoperative level throughout the follow-up. Sociodemographic factors, heavy drinking, and unemployment may be predictive factors of QoL. Still, there is data that claims that surgical treatment, even with free flaps reconstruction, can improve QoL, with direct influence on pain and improvement of diet [27].

In terms of HRQoL, more prospective and multicenter clinical trials should be performed.

3.2 Deglutition rehabilitation

After surgery, the visualization of pharynx is an essential part of a complete examination. Indirect view of the pharynx can be performed with either a mirror or a flexible fiberoptic endoscope. The procedure can be performed when patients are awake, and it is usually well-tolerated. The remaining pharynx can be seen with the mirror and inspected for asymmetry and any potential mucosal abnormalities [28].

Flexible fiberoptic endoscopy can be used for the simple evaluation of the pharynx and also for the assessment of the degree of dysphagia. Dysphagia is a common problem after neck surgery, with an incidence up to 70%, and contributes to compromised nutrition, weight loss which can both lead to diminished quality of life and decreased psychological well-being. Swallowing is a very complex physiological action that is rapid from the beginning to the end [28].

Fiberoptic endoscopic assessment of swallowing (FEES) is a portable procedure that may be completed in outpatient clinic space or at the bedside. FEES involves passing a flexible endoscope through the nose and toward the pharynx to observe swallowing in real-time. FEES is a reliable and sensitive tool for assessing dysphagia [29].

American Speech-Language-Hearing Association (ASHA) states that a clinical-instrumental evaluation of swallowing should reveal: organic and functional alterations in the structures involved, the degree of efficacy of swallowing in its various stages, adequate protection of the lower airways, and coordination between breathing and swallowing. Moreover, it should detect and possibly quantify any penetration of the bolus in the tracheal-bronchial tree. The diagnostic tools used for studying swallowing disorders should be able to assess the various movements that take place during all stages of swallowing in relationship to the type of bolus administered, as well as evaluate the efficacy of the rehabilitation procedures [30, 31].

In spite of the fact that FEES supplies limited information compared to videofluoroscopy because it only investigates the pharyngeal stage followed by a moment of "white-out" in the swallow, it is now employed as a routine procedure. Videoendoscopy permits a static and dynamic evaluation of the structures in the upper airways and upper digestive tract [30, 31].

After the static evaluation of the morphology and function of the upper airways and upper digestive tract, we can also perform a dynamic evaluation of swallowing. For that we administer a bolus to the patient. During the examination, compensatory positions may be kept to improve swallowing efficacy, and also therapeutic maneuvers can be applied in order to establish the appropriate rehabilitation approach for managing, feeding, and swallowing techniques. So, FEES offers the possibility to study the physiology of swallowing, the evaluation of the presence, degree, and type of dysphagia, and is also a good method for establishing the best means of feeding, for advising diets, and for planning any other diagnostic investigation [32].

During FEES we can also use narrow-band imaging (NBI). The optical NBI filter allows a narrow band light with two wavelengths (415 nm blue light and 540 nm green light) to penetrate the tissue to different depths, corresponding to the peaks of absorption of hemoglobin. NBI light is absorbed by vessels but reflected by mucosa, and thus, maximum contrast of vessels and the surrounding mucosa is achieved. Using filtered narrow banded light, pathological epithelial changes are better observed which improves the early detection of dysplasia and carcinoma and allows a better demarcation of benign lesions. Moreover, NBI also helps the assessment of swallowing. It allows better visualization of the bolus and generally leads to much sharper optical contrasts, especially under difficult examination conditions. Consequently, detection of smaller bolus quantities is enhanced and distinction of the bolus from surrounding structures is facilitated [33].

After the assessment of the dysphagia, the rehabilitation plan is determined firstly using postures. The chin-down posture pushes the anterior pharyngeal wall posteriorly, and the tongue base closer to the posterior pharyngeal wall, thus narrowing the airway entrance and reducing aspiration. The head-back posture uses gravity to clear the bolus from the oral cavity and is useful in patients who have difficulty with oral transit of the bolus. Head rotation toward the damaged side of the pharynx closes the damaged side so that the bolus flows down the more-nearly normal side. The lateral head tilt posture may be used for patients who have both unilateral oral and pharyngeal impairment on the same side [34].

In addition to the use of postures, swallow maneuvers may be added. Swallow maneuvers are designed to place specific aspects of the oropharyngeal swallow under voluntary control in order to improve the process. Moreover, some patients may benefit from the modification of bolus size and consistency which may also be effective in eliminating aspiration in patients treated for head and neck cancer. For some patients, a larger volume bolus may be effective at eliciting a more rapid pharyngeal swallow by increasing the sensory input for the patient and so increasing

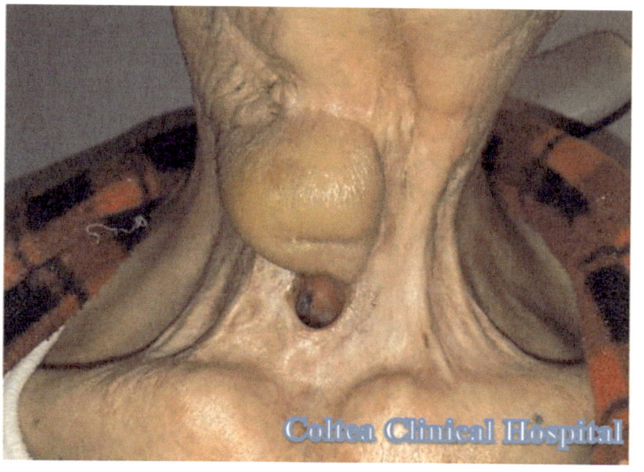

Figure 21.
Free flap reconstruction after fistula complication with vocal prosthesis slightly migrated but with good functional outcome.

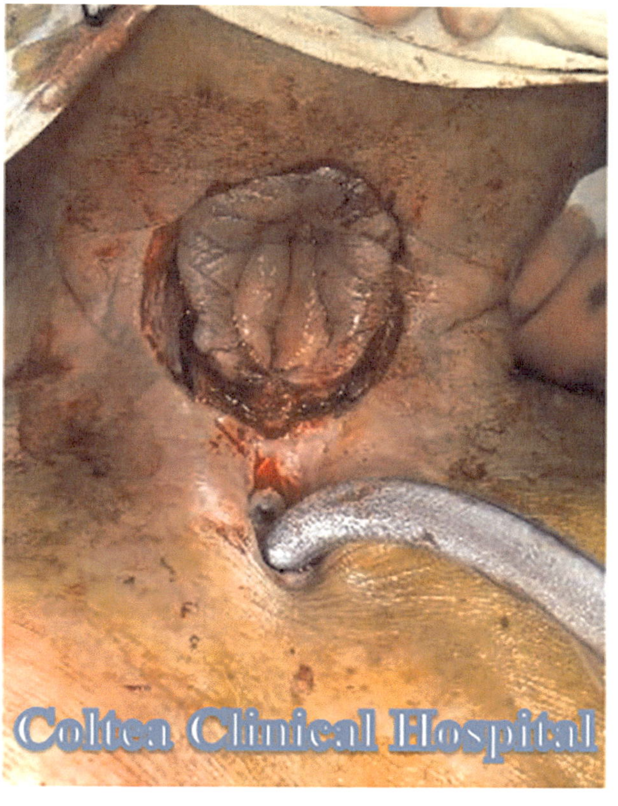

Figure 22.
PMMC reconstruction for fistula complication with vocal prosthesis in place.

awareness of the bolus in the oral cavity. However, patients who require multiple swallows to clear a single bolus will probably benefit from smaller bolus sizes in order to reduce residue and the risk of aspiration [34].

3.3 Voice rehabilitation

Voice rehabilitation is the result of some techniques in which a patient can reach a good functional outcome, with optimal social reinsertion. Voice handicap index, swallowing problems, stoma-related issues, and pain are the most important aspects that can influence QoL index after extensive pharyngeal and laryngeal surgery. Speech therapy, additional nursing care, and patient empowerment may influence the final result after surgery.

After oropharyngeal surgery with primary closure, voice and swallowing may be affected, and the use of radial forearm graft seems to allow a good function. On the other hand, regardless of the way of reconstruction, if the larynx is preserved, the persistence of aspiration/ penetration and consequently the need for a tracheostomy are factors that influence the voice.

After total laryngectomy, with a total separation of the aero-digestive system, air cannot reach higher structures involved in speech, but even though, the neopharynx that is sutured with different techniques can become a neoglottis with sound-producing capacity. Voice rehabilitation after total laryngectomy can be achieved by

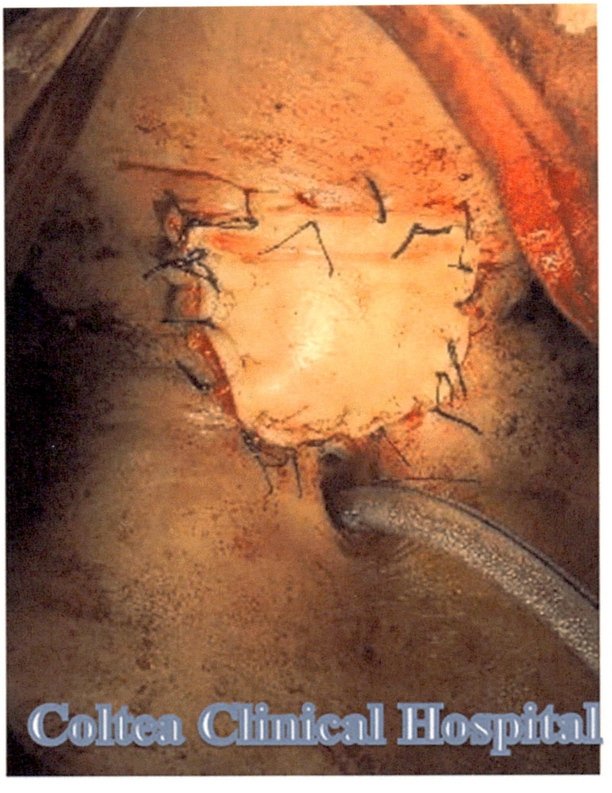

Figure 23.
PMMC reconstruction for fistula complication with vocal prosthesis in place.

esophageal speech (EP), use of an electrolarynx, or tracheoesophageal fistula with a vocal prosthesis (VP).

Tracheoesophageal speech (TES) with VP is the gold standard of voice rehabilitation after total laryngectomy. The main principle of the VP, as a unilateral valve, is that it redirects the exhaled air when the stoma is occluded. As a result, speech is possible as the air reaches the neopharynx, with secondary vibrations, and also the oral cavity. It is a relatively easy to learn technique, with primary placement possibility and low morbidity rates. On the other hand, ES is a difficult-to-learn technique, in which the air is injected with the tongue toward the pharynx and esophagus to make them vibrate. The electrolarynx is a device that produces vibrations and after placing it near the oral cavity, a robotic speech may be achieved.

Hypopharyngeal cancer surgical treatment, even in circular defects and with the need for total reconstruction can now benefit from voice rehabilitation with the use of vocal prosthesis. TES seems to be with good outcome after myofasciocutaneous free flaps and with a lower quality ("wet" or "gurgle" character) after free intestinal flaps. Although some authors claim that after PMMC flap reconstruction a successful TES can be hardly achieved, it has remained a critical reconstructive tool [4, 8] (**Figures 21–23**).

4. Conclusion

The pharynx, as a rendez-vous place of basic physiological and social needs—food intake, breathing, and social interactions, requires a stepped fashion cancer treatment, with a high focus on QoL. Reconstruction is probably one of the most demanding tasks for a head and neck surgeon and often implies a multidisciplinary approach for better outcomes. Keystones after surgery are speech, swallowing, and pulmonary rehabilitation.

Conflict of interest

The authors declare no conflict of interest.

All authors have contributed equally and would like to thank their colleagues for their considerable work and support.

Author details

Paula Luiza Bejenaru[1,2*], Raluca Grigore[1,3], Bogdan Popescu[1,3], Alexandru Nicolaescu[1,4], Mihnea Cojocărița-Condeescu[1,3], Catrinel Simion-Antonie[1,3], Gloria Berteșteanu[1,5], Anca Cirstea[1,3], Teodora Diaconu[1,3], Bianca Taher[1,3], Simona Rujan[1,3], Dan Popescu[1,6] and Șerban V.G. Berteșteanu[1,3]

1 "Carol Davila" University of Medicine and Pharmacy, Bucharest, Romania

2 Dr. Nicolae Kretzulescu" Medical Center for Diagnosis and Ambulatory Treatment, Bucharest, Romania

3 ENT Head and Neck Surgery Clinic, "Colțea" Clinical Hospital, Romania

4 ENT Head and Neck Surgery Compartment, "Prof. Dimitrie Gerota" Emergency Hospital of the Ministry of Internal Affairs, Romania

5 ENT Head and Neck Surgery Clinic, "Dr. Carol Davila" Central Military Hospital, Romania

6 ENT Department, Emergency County Hospital, Targoviste, Romania

*Address all correspondence to: drpaulabejenaru@gmail.com

References

[1] Khaled S. Albahout; Richard A. Lopez. Anatomy, Head and Neck, Pharynx

[2] Dèborados Santos Queija, Juliana Godoy Portas, Rogèrio Aparecido Dedivitis, Carlos Neutzling Lehn, Ana Paula Brandão Barros. Swallowing and quality of life after total laryngectomy and pharyngolaryngectomy

[3] Flint PW, Haughey BH, Lund VJ, Robbins KT, Thomas JR, Lesperance MM, et al. Otolaryngology Head and Neck Surgery. Elsevier Inc; 2021. p. 1401–1422; 1444–1465; 1527–1530

[4] Chu PY, Chang SY. Reconstruction of the hypopharynx after surgical treatment of squamous cell carcinoma. Journal of Chinese Medicine Association. 2009;**72**(7):351-355

[5] Hashim D, Boffetta P. NCCN guidelines: Head and neck cancers. Occupational Cancers. 2020:57-105

[6] Grigore R, Popescu B, Berteşteanu ŞVG, Nichita C, Oașă ID, Munteanu GS, et al. The role of biomaterials in upper digestive tract transoral reconstruction. Materials (Basel). 2021;**14**(6):1-14

[7] Coleman JJ. Reconstruction of the pharynx and cervical esophagus. Seminars in Surgical Oncology. 1995; **11**(3):208-220

[8] Richmon JD, Brumund KT. Reconstruction of the hypopharynx: Current trends. Current Opinion in Otolaryngology & Head and Neck Surgery. 2007;**15**(4):208-212

[9] Sanchez ER, Sanchez R, Moliver C. Anatomic relationship of the pectoralis major and minor muscles: A cadaveric study. Aesthetic Surgery Journal. 2014 Feb;**34**(2):258-263

[10] Solari F, Burns B. Anatomy, Thorax, Pectoralis Major. Treasure Island (FL): StatPearls Publishing; 2022

[11] Tripathi M, Parshad S, Karwasra RK, Singh V. Pectoralis major myocutaneous flap in head and neck reconstruction: An experience in 100 consecutive cases. Natural Journal of Maxillofacial Surgery. 2015;**6**(1):37-41

[12] Burkey B., Futran N. CMF Reconstruction. AO Surgery Refernce [Internet]. 2013. Available from: https://surgeryreference.aofoundation.org/cmf/reconstruction/basic-technique/pectoralis-myocutaneous-pedicle-flap#introduction

[13] Shah J, Snehal P, Bhuvanesh S. Reconostruction with myocutaneous flaps. In: Head and Neck Surgery and Oncology. 4th ed. Elsevier; 2012. pp. 721-728

[14] Akhundzada I, Aliyev A, Huseynov TK, Kerimov RA. Reconstruction of Pharyngeal Defect with Prelaminated Pectoralis Major Pedicled Flap

[15] Jones LF, Farrar EM, Roberts DJH, Moor JW. Revisiting the sternocleidomastoid flap as a reconstructive option in head and neck surgery. The Journal of Laryngology and Otology. 2019;**133**(9):742-746

[16] Bordoni B, Varacallo M. Anatomy, Head and Neck, Sternocleidomastoid Muscle. Treasure Island (FL): StatPearls Publishing; 2022

[17] Clark BS, Shah S. The sternocleidomastoid flap, operative

techniques in otolaryngology. Head and Neck Surgery. 2019;**30**(2):138-144

[18] Eugene N, Myers MD, Snyderman CH. Operative Otolaryngology Head and Neck Surgery. pp. 3768-4178

[19] Nagel TH, Hayden RE. Advantages and limitations of free and pedicled flaps in reconstruction of pharyngoesophageal defects. Current Opinion in Otolaryngology & Head and Neck Surgery. 2014;**22**(5):407-413

[20] Anthony JP, Singer MI, Deschler DG, Dougherty ET, Reed CG, Kaplan MJ. Long-term functional results after pharyngoesophageal reconstruction with the radial forearm free flap. American Journal of Surgery. 1994;**168**:441-445

[21] Disa JJ, Pusic AL, Mehrara BJ. Reconstruction of the hypopharynx with the free jejunum transfer. Journal of Surgical Oncology. 2006;**94**(6):466-470

[22] De Almeida JR, Genden EM. Robotic assisted reconstruction of the oropharynx. Current Opinion in Otolaryngology & Head and Neck Surgery. 2012;**20**(4):237-245

[23] Turner MT, Geltzeiler M, Albergotti WG, Duvvuri U, Ferris RL, Kim S, et al. Reconstruction of TORS oropharyngectomy defects with the nasoseptal flap via transpalatal tunnel. Journal of Robotic Surgery. 2020;**14**(2): 311-316

[24] Aaronson NK, Ahmedzai S, Bergman B, Bullinger M, Cull A, Duez NJ, et al. The European Organisation for Research and Treatment of Cancer QLQ-C30: A quality-of-life instrument for use in international clinical trials in oncology. Journal of the National Cancer Institute. 1993;**85**:365-376

[25] You Q, Jing X, Fan S, Wang Y, Yang Z. Comparison of functional outcomes and health-related quality of life one year after treatment in patients with oral and oropharyngeal cancer treated with three different reconstruction methods. The British Journal of Oral & Maxillofacial Surgery. 2020;**58**(7):759-765

[26] Kim TW, Youm HY, Byun H, Son YI, Baek CH. Treatment outcomes and quality of life in oropharyngeal cancer after Surgery-based versus Radiation-based Treatment. Clinical Experimental in Otorhinolaryngology. 2010;**3**(3):153-160. DOI: 10.3342/ceo.2010.3.3.153

[27] Ma H, Wang XL, Wei MH, An CM. The impact of surgical treatment on the life quality of patients with locally advanced hypopharyngeal carcinoma. Zhonghua Zhong Liu Za Zhi. 2020; **42**(8):687-691

[28] MW Donner, JF Bosma, DL Robertson. Anatomy and physiology of the pharynx

[29] Nicholas Shaheen. Endoscopic Evaluation and Treatment of Swallowing Disorders

[30] Langmore SE, Kenneth SMA, Olsen N. Fiberoptic endoscopic examination of swallowing safety: A new procedure. Dysphagia. 1988;**2**(4): 216-219

[31] A Nacci, F Ursino, R La Vela, F Matteucci, V Mallardi and B Fattori Fiberoptic endoscopic evaluation of swallowing (FEES): Proposal for informed consent

[32] Logemann JA. Swallowing physiology and pathophysiology. Otolaryngologic Clinics of North America. 1988;**21**:613-622

[33] Julie C Nienstedt, Frank Müller, Almut Nießen, Susanne Fleischer, Jana-Christiane Koseki, Till Flügel, Christina Pflug. Narrow Band Imaging Enhances the Detection Rate of Penetration and Aspiration in FEES

[34] Barbara R. Pauloski. Rehabilitation of Dysphagia Following Head and Neck Cancer